Spartan

The Fundamentals of Building Muscle

(A Captivating Guide to the Fierce Warriors of Ancient Greece)

Edwin Elmore

Published By **Darby Connor**

Edwin Elmore

All Rights Reserved

Spartan: The Fundamentals of Building Muscle (A Captivating Guide to the Fierce Warriors of Ancient Greece)

ISBN 978-1-7773611-5-0

No part of this guidebook shall be reproduced in any form without permission in writing from the publisher except in the case of brief quotations embodied in critical articles or reviews.

Legal & Disclaimer

The information contained in this book is not designed to replace or take the place of any form of medicine or professional medical advice. The information in this book has been provided for educational & entertainment purposes only.

The information contained in this book has been compiled from sources deemed reliable, and it is accurate to the best of the Author's knowledge; however, the Author cannot guarantee its accuracy and validity and cannot be held liable for any errors or omissions. Changes are periodically made to this book. You must consult your doctor or get professional medical advice before using any of the suggested remedies, techniques, or information in this book.

Upon using the information contained in this book, you agree to hold harmless the Author from and against any damages, costs, and expenses, including any legal fees potentially resulting from the application of any of the information provided by this guide. This disclaimer applies to any damages or injury caused by the use and application, whether directly or indirectly, of any advice or information presented, whether for breach of contract, tort, negligence, personal injury, criminal intent, or under any other cause of action.

You agree to accept all risks of using the information presented inside this book. You need to consult a professional medical practitioner in order to ensure you are both able and healthy enough to participate in this program.

Table Of Contents

Chapter 1: The Social Structure of Ancient Sparta 1

Chapter 2: Culture and Life in Ancient Sparta 16

Chapter 3: Spartan Military and Battles . 36

Chapter 4: Spartan Helots 44

Chapter 5: The Peloponnesian League and the Fall of Sparta 50

Chapter 6: Famous Spartans 58

Chapter 7: The Spartan Society 67

Chapter 8: The Persian Threat................ 75

Chapter 9: After Thermopylae 105

Chapter 10: Leonidas The Warrior King 128

Chapter 11: The Spartan Legacy........... 137

Chapter 12: the Beginnings of the Spartan Empire 146

Chapter 13: Rise of the Spartan Empire 154

Chapter 14: The Prime of the Spartan Empire 175

Chapter 15: The Fall of the Spartan Empire 181

Chapter 1: The Social Structure of Ancient Sparta

The social shape of historical Sparta is pretty great to that of different metropolis-states within the ancient Greek worldwide. Spartan social shape consisted of 3 social commands – the Spartiates Proper (the elite), the Perioeci (the center magnificence), and the helots (the slaves). When as compared to exclusive Greek city-states, especially Athens, there has been now not a whole lot of a divide some of the Spartiates Proper and the Perioeci, or maybe the helot magnificence, the slaves of the alternative commands, had an prolonged way more freedom and benefits than slaves a few vicinity else inside the historic international. The Spartiates Proper and the Perioeci have been extra concerned with military training and advancing their competencies than surrounding themselves with luxuries. The ancient Spartans have been well-known for shelling out their wealth, and so dealt with their social education a protracted way in any other manner than what the Athenians did, making the Spartan social shape unique.

Men and Women in Ancient Sparta

Women in the ancient Greek global had been at the entire predicted to stay at domestic and be subservient better halves tending to the home and children. Spartan girls were virtually as sturdy as Spartan guys; each sexes informed from an early age and expected to be bodily healthy. Neither gender became allowed to fail and training and exercising training began out in formative years for each.

The Spartiates Proper

The Spartiates Proper become the social elite and loved whole Spartan citizenship. Their numbers had been not as excessive due to the fact the Perioeci or the helots, however they were furnished with many advantages the others didn't. Much in their lives had been targeted on advancing their navy capabilities and maintaining physical health. In addition to this, they may vote on political subjects and could personal helots to art work their land. Spartiates Proper have been not anticipated to do guide labour and at the same time as they had been the social elite, their lives have been extremely precise to the social elite a few place else.

The Perioeci

The Periocei had been the second one beauty residents, or the middle beauty, of historic Sparta. Those who belonged to this social beauty loved certain blessings – along with unfastened motion internal and out of Sparta, to very personal land, emerge as hoplites and enrol within the navy – however they have been no longer complete citizens and couldn't be a part of in on political subjects or marry a Spartiate Proper.

The Helots

The helots had been basically the slaves of historical Sparta and the bottom class. Archaeologists don't forget that when the

Spartans defeated the Messenians, they delivered a number of them yet again to Laconia to function slaves. While the helots were better handled than excellent slaves in historic Greece, they resented the Spartans and rose up in the direction of their masters numerous times at some point of the centuries. The helots had been authorized to live in their personal houses, raising their non-public families and saved part of the vegetation they tended for his or her proprietors but were no longer authorized to be sociable with the Spartiates Proper.

When looking at Sparta in evaluation to Athens and distinct locations in ancient Greece, it's far clean that the social shape of this town-country changed into pretty smooth however first rate. The social elite, whilst taking element in diverse blessings, did no longer stay a lifestyles of high-priced in evaluation to different elite organizations and the bottom of the low, the helots, lived better existence than others of the same elegance, resulting in historical Sparta owning one of the maximum unique social systems visible in the historic global.

The Spartan Elders

Also referred to as the Gerousia, the Spartan Elders consisted of the two Spartan kings and 30 men who met the set requirements. Only Spartiates Proper guys over the age of 60 might also want to apply to be an Elder, and people who had more noble blood or social fame had higher odds of becoming a member of.

The Gerousia held high-quality power and importance in Spartan society. They had been able to be worried in politics and act because the middleman between the kings and the other Spartans. They had been additionally able to choose out residents within the Spartan court docket, preserving the power to exile and punish folks that had committed crimes.

Spartan Women

Spartan women have been required to be each bodily and mentally strong. Along with boys, women have been informed from an early age, reading approximately the arts, facts, philosophy, music, battle and different subjects. Spartan girls held an extended manner greater energy and dealt with more similarly than Greek girls a few extraordinary region. But regardless of the more freedoms that that they had, a Spartan lady still had to fulfil a effective role, surely as men had to.

Health of Spartan Women

Spartan girls were anticipated to be both bodily and mentally healthy. It became believed that handiest robust, healthy girls have to supply begin to sturdy, healthful youngsters. Women have been, therefore, required to participate in regular workout training, some aspect quite first rate among remarkable Greek women of the day.

The Advantages

Sparta girls loved severa distinct blessings that exceptional Greek women did not. In Athens and specific city-states, women had been best approved a sure quantity to devour. In evaluation, Spartan ladies have been allowed to eat what they desired and drink wine in fact as a good buy as Spartan guys. Although not referred to for first-rate, it's miles believed that they've been allowed to eat and drink as an awful lot as they wanted due to the fact they burned extra energy due to exercise often.

Marriage

Women in Sparta did not count on to marry till she end up in her overdue teens or early twenties, over again, some problem pretty one-of-a-kind to that of ladies a few place else. Most girls married in their early young adults within the historic international, so for a Spartan female marrying so late in existence, it come to be considered pretty unusual.

However, it moreover had a few different advantage – childbirth. Spartan girls were sturdy and in flip, believed with a purpose to giving starting to robust children. This became the principle cause why girls married despite the fact that couples did now not stay together for some time after the wedding. It became believed that with the useful resource of living aside, the bond should reinforce a number of the couple.

A traditional marriage amongst Spartan couples modified into basically what have become said in historic times as a 'captured marriage'. The bride's maid of honour or her bridesmaids could capture her, reduce off her hair in reality and then dress her in guys's apparel. The groom would leave his mess corridor and they'll start a secret marriage together. The couple might also need to fulfill in mystery till the character have come to be thirty.

Motherhood

A robust girl makes a strong guy, it end up stated. Spartan guys were stated to be sturdy because of their mothers. Loyalty to the Sparta changed into emphasised from an early age. Children have been dealt with almost similarly in Sparta, with boys staying of their mother's houses till they have been seven years old after which taken to the barracks to start navy training. Girls should live with their mothers until they married.

For Spartan girls, being a mother have turn out to be the number one feature in society. The helots would probably work the land in order that women should provide attention to motherhood and supply beginning to strong kids who could in all likelihood shield Sparta.

Women in Sparta were unlike another Greek girls — they were strong, relatively knowledgeable, might probable learn how to war and fight and teach her children, male and lady, to do the same. Enjoying freedoms, schooling and plenty of numerous advantages, it become simplest possible for a female to live this manner in Sparta.

Children of Sparta

From transport, Spartan youngsters were required to be robust. Life modified into tough in Sparta and fine the fittest, the maximum effective, youngsters have to live on. Children had been predicted to develop as lots as defend Sparta and fine the strong, rapid and smartest must address that duty.

Spartan youngsters underwent several tests developing up, the first one accomplished surely after start. Sparta only had use for the most effective and if a little one seemed ill or awful, they have been abandoned out of doors the metropolis, typically close to the mountains. If wild animals didn't kill the babies, then the factors did. Sparta had little need for sick youngsters.

Every Spartan toddler, whether boy or woman, became tested at shipping. Infant boys have been washed in wine, a concept believed to offer them energy sufficient to prepare for their destiny army training. When we observe how children had been treated, it's miles clean that Spartan kids had been treated similarly – all had to be physical and mentally sturdy to protect and serve the dominion and all and sundry had the possibility to reveal this all through their lifetimes.

Spartan Girls

Spartan women should live with their mom till they married, however may additionally want to begin their schooling at spherical seven years antique. Education for girls turned into taken considerably in Sparta, a idea no longer shared a few vicinity else inside the historic Greek global, and prefer Spartan boys, the women could in all likelihood exercise and be educated in a fixed.

It isn't always completely clean as to what Spartan women learnt but it's also popular that they learnt similar subjects to Spartan boys. This covered the humanities, song, philosophy, facts, drama, analyzing, writing and poetry. It come to be specific to Sparta girls as nowhere else in the historic Greek international might girls take shipping of such training.

Girls in Sparta had been expected to be honestly as physically in shape as the boys. Only bodily robust ladies should amplify up and supply begin to strong, healthy youngsters. Spartan girls may want to workout with the lads outside, every exceptional precise element in their manner of lifestyles in evaluation to extraordinary Greek women who weren't even allowed out of doors the house until despatched on an errand. Spartan women would have a look at gymnastics, wrestling and combat skills – all of which might be used to protect Sparta or themselves if faced with the state of affairs.

When ladies have become 18 years antique they confronted the subsequent predominant test and will want all their bodily training in case you need to bypass and benefit complete

Spartan citizenship. Whilst it isn't always positive what the take a look at covered, it is believed it become a mixture of bodily and mental bodily sports, allowing them to show their capabilities. If the woman surpassed, she modified into grated whole Spartan citizenship but if she failed then she would possibly take delivery of the rank of perioikos, successfully turning into center beauty. Whether she exceeded or not, after the of completion of the test she have emerge as a citizen and loved all the advantages that got here with it.

Spartan Boys

After boys had passed the number one check they then wished to expose themselves worth of being a Spartan and capable of defending the kingdom. Until they had been six or seven, boys might stay at the circle of relatives home (commonly with their parents or their mother and her servants if her husband changed into however living within the barracks or had died) however from start they might had been knowledgeable that defensive the us of a modified into above the whole lot else.

Training in Childhood

Upon leaving the circle of relatives home, Spartan boys might bypass into the navy barracks with extraordinary boys their very personal age to start their education, becoming a part of the Agoge. State education modified into divided into three elements primarily based absolutely mostly on age; the primary starting at six or seven to 17, the second between 17 and 20 years antique, and the 0.33 from 20 to 29/30 years, which proper now Spartan men have been allowed to transport out of the barracks and have been given extra rights as a Spartan citizen.

In the second one a part of their training (amongst 17 and two decades vintage), they had been now not classed as guys however have been mechanically enrolled in the navy as reserves. They could nice pass into warfare if and at the same time as the situation referred to as for it. They can also be a part of the secret police or be delegated as part of a very specific defend.

The zero.33 segment started when they have turn out to be 20 and had been voted into considered one of numerous public messes. Those already in the messes should decide who become voted in. It is thought that boys had up to 10 years to earn the right to sign up for one of the messes.

Life for Spartan youngsters have come to be now not smooth regardless of how antique they had been. From begin till maturity, they had to prove themselves well worth of being Spartan. This intended you needed to be healthful, physical robust and mentally capable otherwise you were no longer going to live on, whether or not or not you were a boy or a woman.

Chapter 2: Culture and Life in Ancient Sparta

Life in Sparta became difficult. Military education started out at a greater younger age and persevered nicely into adulthood. However, it changed into not the quality part of historic Spartan lifestyle and life-style.

Food and Diet

Food and food plan in Sparta become confined to what have become to be had within the neighborhood location. Whereas citizenships from a few location else in Greece enjoyed meals, the Spartan weight loss plan modified right into a good buy extra fundamental and modest.

The Spartans noticed meals as a technique to an cease. Food changed proper into a want, a manner of staying wholesome and sturdy on the way to protect the u . S .. It have become no longer essential to over-take pride in food as extraordinary city-states did as it'd have a bad impact on their physical schooling, some factor that could not be tolerated in Spartan society.

The majority of the meals that changed into placed in Spartan diets changed into produced via the helots grown on their grasp's lands. The maximum common food decided in Spartan diets blanketed milk, cheese, honey, bread, figs, sparkling quit result, wine and meat from a whole lot of tremendous animals.

Whilst Spartans were particularly professional as warriors, they have been exceptional hunters. Any animal changed into used as a meals deliver however also supplied them a way of recreation and education workout. No part of the animal killed might be wasted. Sheep, goats and pigs had been the principle belongings of meat, in addition to fish at the same time as it changed into available. Wild boar, rabbits and special wild animals can be eaten after a a hit hunt.

Dairy changed proper right into a primary staple in the Spartan healthy eating plan, with the milk taken from nearby goats and sheep used to make cream and cheese. The Spartans had been well-known for their cheeses all through Greece. Bread have become moreover eaten in Sparta even though it wasn't a large a part of their eating regimen. Instead of using wheat to make bread, the Spartans used barley, however may additionally use the former on particular sports.

Black broth, or black soup, is assumed to had been the number one meals dish in Sparta however the fact that a number of historical sources claim it wasn't that commonplace. However, it's far the most acquainted of all of the Spartan dishes. Black broth modified into stated to were made with boiled red meat, vinegar, salt and blood.

Wine changed into enjoyed in Sparta however, as with everything else, some thing now not be over-indulged in. Wine became beneath the have an effect on of alcohol with or after the majority of food however modified into usually watered down while you recollect that being under the influence of alcohol have grow to be frowned upon. The Spartans believed that being under the effect of alcohol had a negative impact on each the body and the thoughts, creating a soldier susceptible and therefore incapable of protective Sparta.

The Spartan mindset in the direction of food and wine turn out to be clearly just like different components – food was crucial to keep one bodily healthy and strong. A Spartan might not take pride in meals and wine because of the bad consequences. In this manner, the Spartan weight loss plan changed into pretty healthy, even by means of manner of in recent times's standards.

Entertainment in Sparta

Whilst the Spartans had been devoted to progressing their military skills, they did have a number of considered one of a type pursuits after they weren't education. The Spartans took terrific pleasure of their hobbies, giving them as plenty self-discipline and focus as they did in the route of their physical training. It didn't remember variety whether or not it emerge as searching, dancing or taking element in a competition – the Spartans were a humans that have been devoted to a few factor they centered their minds on.

Athletics

Athletics have end up a huge part of Spartan life. Everyone might take part in athletics – man, girl, boy, lady extra younger or vintage – and the beyond-time became an vital element of Sparta's photo. Women have been recommended to participate, a few element in evaluation to women some location else in Greece, and they have been notably right at it. When no longer involved in battle, Spartans may want to experience in this, becoming so right that they regularly competed in opposition to extraordinary Greek metropolis-states within the Olympic Games and others, triumphing numerous.

Dancing

Dancing emerge as a well-known hobby in Sparta. It become a amusing hobby and because the Spartans had no problems regarding their our our bodies, dancing allowed them to have fun and display off their physical abilties off the education area. Dancing have become achieved at celebrations and gala's which included the Gymnopaedia which became held on an annual basis.

Hunting

Hunting become each a interest and a opposition in Sparta. When there had been no battles available, looking allowed Spartan warriors to keep their abilties sharp further to presenting them with the an awful lot wanted uncooked substances which consist of wood, food and animal skins. A tremendous Spartan hunt blanketed horses, the lakonian hounds and the helots to hold any animals caught. For the Spartan hunter, the kills have been a competition amongst them and the animal in question and kills had been made up close.

Banquets

The Spartans did now not take pride in lavish portions of food and wine but have to preserve banquets at unique sports and festivals. There were numerous festivals celebrated in Sparta, which incorporates the Hyacinthia, held in honour of Hyacinthus, a divine hero whose cult come to be held at Amyclae in Sparta. A big dinner party grow to be held on the second one day of his party as well as developing a music, horse racing and distinct occasions.

Sparta modified right into a military u . S ., with its citizens raised to be physical and mentally strong however the Spartans used numerous interests and interests to hold on excelling their our bodies with bodily sports activities even as playing themselves.

Religion in Sparta

Just with the opposite Greek city-states, the Spartans believed in masses of gods. At the time Sparta rose to great energy, Zeus and the opportunity Olympian gods have been the principle deities worshipped in Greece, with Zeus main the pantheon.

Sparta became a deeply religious nation and their strong determination to the gods become regularly mocked via other Greek states. While others gave the gods their due worship and no more, the Spartans submitted and revered the gods with out query.

The ancient Greek gods had been worshipped in the direction of the u . S . A ., with each metropolis and town-nation often devoted to at least one deity especially. Sparta changed into simply much like the alternative Greek town-states. For instance, in Sparta, Aphrodite changed into a popular goddess. Throughout the rest of ancient Greece, Aphrodite grow to be referred to as the goddess of physical love, but in Sparta she emerge as considered a goddess of warfare, which have become apt due to the fact the Spartans were a warrior race and taken into consideration girls to be more identical to guys than everywhere else in Greece.

Favourite Gods

The Spartans had severa gods which they worshipped specially others. These blanketed Aphrodite, Ares (the god of conflict) and Apollo (the god of prophecy and looking, amongst others), all of whom had tendencies which corresponded to the Spartans navy way of existence. However, the Spartans worshipped all of the gods and held severa gala's in the route of the 12 months of their honour.

Religious Festivals

Although Sparta turn out to be within the most important a military united states, they held several religious celebrations. The Hyacinthia (moreover spelt Hyakinthia) became really one in all the most important spiritual sports activities in Sparta, held over three days and emerge as devoted to Hyacinthus a divine hero, and the god Apollo.

Held in early summer time, the primary day become devoted to mourning the lack of life of the hero, with a sombre dinner party held in his honour. The 2nd day became to have amusing his rebirth with song, dancing and horse races. The 1/three day turned into sombre, with the women weaving a chiton and providing it to the gods.

The Gymnopaedia have become held in the summer season and come to be held in honour of Apollo and several different deities. In this competition, naked youths ought to display their physical and athletic abilities and carry out warfare dances and musical abilities.

The Enyalia turn out to be a competition where the Spartans may sacrifice a canine to the god Enyalius, who may be taken into consideration a manifestation of the god Ares.

The Carnea (or Karneia) pageant turned into some other as a substitute popular competition held in Sparta. It emerge as dedicated to Apollo Carneus, the god of the flocks, herds and the harvest, in which single youths might also need to chase a man (probable a clergyman in the company to the god). If the man or woman grow to be caught, then it supposed that the metropolis is probably wealthy. If he wasn't caught, the city wouldn't be. The Carnea pageant have become so famous that battles had been postponed in order that they wouldn't be interrupted. In reality, it emerge as said that the handiest motive why Leonidas marched to war with three hundred squaddies have become because the relaxation have been celebrating Carnea at the time and he did no longer want to offend the gods.

Spartan Priests

Whilst the Spartans had been committed to the gods, they did not have any set priests. In fact, the closest thing they needed to clergymen were the kings themselves. The kings had been believed to be the clergymen of Zeus, the king of the gods, and in order that they took at the function of priest in Spartan faith, performing as an middleman between the gods and men.

Religion modified into part of Spartan life, honestly because it have become anywhere else in Greece. The gods worshipped in Sparta have been many, with Zeus considered to be the pleasant of all of them. Many goddesses have been seen as conflict-like, which corresponded with the view that ladies must be truely as physically and mentally robust as Spartan guys. Of course, being a military country, the Spartans favoured robust, warfare-like gods consisting of Ares and Apollo, but every god became worshipped and revered in Sparta.

Spartan Architecture

Sparta become extra concerned approximately their physical capabilities and their electricity than they were approximately their structure. The Spartan mind-set end up approximately defence in place of artwork, and their shape presentations this fantastic.

Buildings in Sparta were stark, hardy and useful pretty else.

Whilst Sparta turned into one of the most effective metropolis-states, it wasn't without a doubt what may be taken into consideration a city itself. Athens, as an instance, became a metropolis contained and protected by means of the use of a massive wall. Sparta, instead, changed into an entire lot greater open than Athens, not covered through a wall or a few element else to protect it like exceptional cities. One of the crucial motives for this become that the Spartans navy might grow to be both professional and feared during Greece, and city-kingdom leaders should no longer march on Sparta with out thinking times on it. Not most effective this, however Sparta's place in the Laconia place gave it a diploma of natural safety from their enemies.

Family Homes

Sparta has always been referred to as a robust, army civilization but the majority of the country have turn out to be farmland.

Farming has commonly been a tough way of life and so the standard Spartan circle of relatives home contemplated this. Spartan houses have been usually one diploma, notwithstanding the fact that may be levels immoderate as had been the norm some vicinity else inside the Greek worldwide, and had been produced from solar-dried dust bricks. The roof would possibly have consisted of purple clay tiles and the residence might probable have had a courtyard inside the centre. Houses have been painted white that permits you to reflect the heat and keep the residence cool.

Spartan Barracks

Spartan boys lived in navy barracks from the age of six or seven to start their valid training. No Spartan barracks has been unearthed however archaeologists trust that they have been very much like that during their own family homes, just more clean interior, in addition to army barracks discovered some other location in Greece. The barracks are presumed to be square with a extensive courtyard, or U-shaped with an open courtyard to the rear. The courtyards must have featured a roofed walkway, imparting shade for the ones not engaged inside any interest.

Helot Houses

The helots were basically the serfs of the Spartans but had been given far extra freedoms than everyone else in ancient Greece. The helots had been typical to have their very very personal residences however had been a ways simpler than that of the Spartans homes.

The Theatre

The ancient theatre is one in every of the maximum critical and maximum critical Spartan homes to have survived the a long term. It changed into built around 25 BCE to seat extra than 15,000 Spartans with Mount Taygetus supplying a lovable backdrop. In the second century CE Pausanias defined it as:

"this theatre fabricated from white stone is sight worth".

The majority of Spartan homes have sadly been misplaced to us over the past 2,000 years. As a end end result, lots of our information on Spartan form is critically limited. From what we recognize of the Spartans attitude, they did not over-take delight in many things, who determine upon a smooth and stark manner of existence, and their form most probable pondered this.

Clothing

As with distinct components of the Spartan manner of lifestyles, garb changed into clean and slight. The Spartans may be classed as warriors who lived farming lifestyles and as a surrender result, their clothing have become smooth and essential. However, the Spartans had a love of shiny purple and will be worn as they went into struggle. Colours were believed to be woman with red being the least feminine out of they all. In addition to this, pink clothing hid blood stains simpler and consequently must mislead their enemies that they weren't harmed in any respect.

Tunics/Chitons

The tunic, additionally known as the chiton, changed into the maximum popular piece of garb in Sparta. It consisted of a massive square piece of material which become then wrapped throughout the frame and stored in area via pins and buttons. The Spartan chitons were maximum likely similar to that of the tunics worn with the aid of way of various Greeks. In the summer season, they may probable have worn lighter material probable made via the girls or helots and within the wintry climate, replaced by heavier woollen chitons. However, a few assets have said that the selection of fabric was due to the term in vicinity of via the season itself.

Footwear

Spartans can also need to have picks at the same time as it came to footwear – every sandals or boots. Sandals have been open-toed and made from leather-based totally in a clean layout, with the Laconian boot moreover open-toed and simple which will allow the wearer to transport much less tough or to account for the hotter climate.

Cloaks

When we see depictions of Spartan warriors in war we commonly see them sporting their iconic pink cloaks. This photo is usually a rely of wonderful argument amongst students as it's far difficult to recognize why a Spartan warrior should put on a cloak into war even as it is able to encumber him. There are many students who be given as real with they did placed on them, even within the middle of the battlefield, as it gave them steady haven and warmth, specially after they had been stopping in cold regions.

The himation and the chlamys were the 2 maximum famous forms of cloaks within the ancient Greek international, worn each the Spartans and one-of-a-type Greeks. In many depictions of Spartan warriors, they will be shown sporting the chlamys, with the cloak draped over the shoulder. The himation cloak have end up worn over every shoulders. The Spartans are believed to have worn the chlamys cloak each day at the identical time as wanted and changed into dyed purple.

Women's Clothes

Spartan women, like different Greek women, may normally placed on a chiton despite the fact that they may wear a shorter version, most probably due to the reality longer patterns ought to get in their way while education and exercising. Elsewhere inside the Greek worldwide, Spartan ladies have been often gossiped approximately for sporting more risqué clothing than themselves.

Helot Clothing

The helots had been given plenty extra freedoms than serfs some different place in historical Greece however the helots were not allowed to dress just like that of the

Spartans. The restricted facts we've were given on the helots garb is that their garb emerge as easy and that they wore leather-based-based-based totally caps as to suggest their repute.

The garb worn with the beneficial aid of the Spartans changed into very similar to that of various elements in their lives – clean and useful. The Spartans desired to transport naked on the same time as they'll – an entire lot to the wonder of the relaxation of the Greek world – however it is probably because garments had been given within the way of their training. However, while their regular garb have become easy and undeniable in coloration, at the same time as it came to battle they wore an impressive blood-pink cloak which is probably resultseasily stated from afar, putting terror into the hearts in their enemies.

Chapter 3: Spartan Military and Battles

The Spartan army changed into one of the most powerful and most effective the historic international has ever stated. Spartan warriors were feared a protracted way and big, and the mere idea of going thru them on the battlefield brought about distinct Greek armies to shake. The Spartan military became sturdy and fearsome because of the reality that they have been raised navy-style from a very young age in order that after they have been vintage enough, they can be part of the army and shield the us of a.

The Spartan Military and Its Ideals

Life in the Spartan army come to be tough. From childhood to adulthood, warriors needed to be bodily and mentally strong, but additionally they had a strict identity which allowed them to combat in a way the ancient global had in no manner visible earlier than. Together, status as a fixed, they had been ambitious.

Code of Honour

The Spartans had been not handiest recognized for his or her fierce preventing capabilities however their strength of mind to a strict code of honour. This code of honour modified into the important aspect to their success and that they face grave dishonour in the event that they didn't live through it. The code of honour protected severa factors which covered how they acted every on and off the battlefield. In war, a Spartan warrior had to act in a way that didn't get his fellow soldier damage. Warriors had to make certain that they acted flippantly in conflict, even when the battlefield turned into in chaos, for the motive that recklessness ought to harm the relaxation of the phalanx. Warriors may on occasion talk and pass in gradual, calculated steps within the course of the enemy. If they broke a long way from the phalanx, not caring about the relaxation of the business enterprise, it changed into feasible that they may be banished from Sparta and now not be a Spartan citizen.

The Spartan Navy

The Spartans have been not identified for his or her love of the ocean and the bulk in their forces may be located on land. However, the Spartans however maintained a small naval fleet at a few diploma in the Persian Wars which then grew more potent in later years. However, the Spartan military changed into eventually defeated through the Athenians and the Persians running together.

Military Campaigns

The battles and wars which the Spartans engaged in have end up legends subsequently of the centuries. Although the Spartans preferred to battle near home, there had been instances after they had to adventure lengthy distances to combat. Marching lengthy distances come to be now not some problem the Spartans have been fans of and would often refuse to take part in battles if marching a long way from domestic was required. Although the Spartans did not have any incredible military techniques as compared to that of the other Greek warriors of the time, their willpower to refining their capabilities made them fantastically professional.

Spartan Battles

The Spartans were engaged in severa battles over the centuries which led them to being referred to as one of the most effective states in Greece by means of the fifth century BCE. The earliest wars they have been concerned in have been the Messenian Wars at some stage within the 7th and 6th centuries BCE, the Argive Wars maximum of the 6th and fourth centuries BCE, and the Arcadian and Megaran Wars at some stage in the 5th and fourth centuries BCE.

The Messenian Wars

The Messenian Wars started out in 743 BCE and lasted for two decades. The Spartans preferred greater land and in the end conquered the Messenians regardless of having fewer infantrymen than their enemy. Their diffused navy competencies allowed them to seize the Messenians and bring them decrease returned to Sparta as their serfs, farming the land for Sparta. The Messenians, but, did no longer like this and in the long run revolted in the course in their masters around forty years later. The 2d Messenian War lasted for 17 years and all another time, the Messenians were defeated by using manner of using the Spartans.

The Persian Wars

For just over 50 years, the Persian Empire tried to take manage of Greece and there have been severa battles which came about most of the Greek metropolis-states and the Persians. However, the vital battle changed into held at Thermopylae in 480 BCE wherein King Leonidas of Sparta defended a slender pass in opposition to the Persians at Thermopylae with just three hundred men. The Spartans were sooner or later defeated due to the fact the majority of the Spartan warriors refused to march up to now a long way from Sparta.

The Peloponnesian War

In the 5th century BCE, the two largest states had been Sparta and Athens who were sour fighters. Athens and the Delian League joined forces to create the Peloponnesian League which then raged struggle on Sparta. The first battle among the 2 forces started out round 431 BCE and endured for 3 many years. The end result was that Sparta destroyed Athens and took her location due to the fact the strongest energy of the day. However, it wasn't clearly Athens that suffered – numerous extraordinary Greek towns have been destroyed and suffered significantly at some stage in this time.

Battle of Leuktra

One of the critical thing battles in Spartan data grow to be the conflict of Leuktra among Thebes and Sparta. Taking region in July 371 BCE on the plain ofLeuctra (close to present day Levktra) in southern Boeotia, wherein Thebes, Athens and distinctive Greek cities faced Sparta. Known because of the fact the

Boeotian League and led through Thebes, the wars carried on with nobody side triumphing. Eventually, peace talks had been noted but because of the reality not all the representatives for the Boeotian League arrived to sign the report, Sparta did now not comply with it. The war began once more, and in the long run the Spartans have been defeated. It became dropping this struggle which prompted the Spartans dying and at the identical time as they did live to inform the story, they now not wielded the energy they as fast as had.

The Spartans relished conflict but did no longer enjoy being too a protracted way far from home to have interaction in it. Their love of home brought on them to refuse to enter conflict on numerous sports. Their enemies were all too privy to the power the Spartans possessed however on uncommon sports, they showed they, too, have been sincerely human and the struggle of Leuktra marked the prevent of the terrific Spartan electricity.

Retirement from the Army

After a Spartan man reached the age of 60, he turned into able to retire from military existence. He not needed to train nor did he must go to war if a warfare have become known as and will be part of the Gerousia.

Chapter 4: Spartan Helots

The helots had been the serfs, or slaves, of historic Sparta. The helots have been the lowest of the all of the instructions and had been used by the Spartans to paintings the farms and exceptional jobs. Scholars be given as real with that the Spartans captured the Messenians within the seventh century BCE to farm their land so they will address their physical education.

Studies on the Spartans normally have a propensity to reputation at the warriors themselves but the helots have been an essential a part of Spartan society. The helots should now not exceptional will be inclined to the land, make apparel and prepare meals, however may moreover march to war with the Spartans if and even as it modified into vital. The helots lived in a metropolis-nation wherein they may moreover work their way out of their lowly class thru severa ways, which incorporates showing exceptional bravery at the battlefield or being relatively honest.

Understanding the Helots

The foundation for the meaning of the phrase helots is shrouded in thriller however the most commonplace belief is that it derives from the village of Helos, positioned to the south of Sparta in which the primary slaves had been considering the useful useful resource of Sparta.

The Beginning

The First Messenian War started out out in 743 BCE and continued for the following 20 years with the Spartans claiming victory over the Messenians. Those Messenians who were no longer able to flee were now proclaimed helots, slaves to Sparta. For the Messenians who have been now not able to break out their new masters, their youngsters should now be born into slavery, serving Sparta's dreams. However, the helots have to fast outnumber the Spartans and would upward thrust up closer to them severa times over the subsequent couple of centuries.

How Were the Helots Were Treated?

Slaves may be decided inside the direction of historical Greece however Sparta had an extraordinarily tolerant mindset within the path of theirs. The helots have been handled a long way more kindly in Sparta, given severa advantages and freedoms, than their opposite numbers acquired a few vicinity else. For example, even as the helots had been required to farm the land and bring the vegetation had to keep the kingdom, they had been general to keep an great a part of the flora for themselves. It has been predicted that they'll get maintain of nearly half of the flowers yielded.

The helots had been moreover allowed to marry and to elevate youngsters. Elsewhere in Greece, the lives of the slaves were tightly controlled and had been no longer allowed to breed as speedy because the helots have been accepted. Because of this, the helots variety fast swelled and overtook the Spartans. They furthermore had their very own homes, could purchase their very own land and will maintain their personal traditions, languages and extremely good freedoms.

The helots have been moreover quite fortunate inside the fact that they'll paintings their manner out of their lowly caste. Some helots can also need to upward thrust in reputation to what modified into referred to as Neodamodeis, which interprets as "made one of the network". In this, helots who had demonstrated themselves on the battlefield or had come what might also gained enough repute could take transport of this perceive. We do no longer realise for superb what they received from this marketing however it is idea they were able to get hold of greater jobs have been be given as actual with have emerge as essential as they carried on walking their way in the direction of freedom.

Helot Rebellions

While the helots enjoyed great freedoms under Spartan rule, they have been however serfs and controlled. They bided their time, their distaste for being servants to their conquerors simmering beneath the floor, till they ultimately rebelled and attempted to regain their freedom.

The first helot upward thrust up in competition to Sparta is called the Second Messenian War. It is normally regular that this warfare commenced round 685 BCE and in the end concluded in 668 BCE with the Argives supporting the Messenian helots in their conflict. However, it wasn't enough and the Spartans had been effective.

Aristomenes

Aristomenes changed proper right into a Messenian hero who has been in big thing ascribed the function of the chief of the helots or maybe accrediting him with beginning the Second Messenian War. He managed to win several victories all through the struggle however modified into betrayed with the beneficial useful resource of King Aristocrates of Arcadia who had formerly supported him. For 11 years, Aristomenes became besieged in Eira till the Spartans in the end took control of it and captured him. He have become exiled to Rhodes wherein he in the end died.

The Third Revolt

The helots had been sooner or later capable of win their freedom round 370 – 350 BCE even as Sparta have emerge as inclined after stopping closer to the Peloponnesian League currently. The Messenians have been in the end freed via Epaminodas of Thebes, in spite of the truth that the helot device persisted on until the second one century BCE.

Chapter 5: The Peloponnesian League and the Fall of Sparta

The Spartans confronted many adversaries at a few level within the centuries. From the earliest instances, in particular after the Messenian Wars, Sparta had all commenced out to stamp their mark on Greek facts and their dominance over the u . S . A .. As a prevent cease end result, many different city-states warred upon them, hoping to be the only to defeat them. Greece become to be a rustic constantly at warfare. In order to preserve stability, the Peloponnesian League turned into long-established.

The Peloponnesian League have become an alliance of metropolis-states from the Peloponnese region and changed into based totally through Sparta itself. It have become created with a view to determined a strong relationship maximum of the town-states inside the area a exquisite manner to maintain peace and safety. The Spartans every desired to keep their vicinity of shipping steady from threats and had been organized to revenue struggle to achieve this, but on the equal time moreover they preferred peace. The Peloponnesian League changed into primarily based totally to maintain this, sponsored up with the may of several states in a global regularly besieged with battle.

The Beginning of the Peloponnesian League

The Peloponnesian League, additionally called the Spartan Alliance, started out to take vicinity with the turn of the 6th century BCE at the equal time because the ancient international was starting to recognize Sparta's electricity. At this time, the Messenians were completely defeated and the Delian League have been long-established with the aid of the usage of Athens. The Delian League have end up an alliance of towns who have been promised safety from the Persians. Because of this, Sparta counteracted with the Peloponnesian League.

The Foundation of the Peloponnesian League

Formed in the sixth century BCE, the Peloponnesian League end up unique on the time Cleomenes I become king of Sparta and took a leading characteristic in its creation. The Delian League had spurred the Spartans and King Cleomenes to do so, to create a league that could rival the Athenian-led Delian League need to they, or every distinctive town-america, now not be given as actual with the Athenians and for that reason ordinary their private solidity.

The Delian League vs. The Peloponnesian League

There had been some of versions the various Delian and the Peloponnesian Leagues. The Delian League, named after its financial organization on the island of Delos, charged an admission fee to all who needed to sign up in even as the Peloponnesian League didn't rate. A kind of metropolis-states were not happy with this membership fee and the Spartans used this whilst it came to putting in place their private league. The Spartans also gave all people a unmarried vote each, irrespective of how large their u . S . Turn out to be. In this, then, the Peloponnesian League have come to be fairer to its people than what the Athenians had been with the Delian League.

However, all individuals have been required to contribute one 1/3 in their navy to the Peloponnesian League when they went to war. Again, there was an detail of fairness on this proviso due to the truth that no one state had to sacrifice their complete navy and they will nevertheless decorate a powerful military if and at the same time as the need arose.

The Necessity of the Peloponnesian League

Sparta and Athens had prolonged been combatants and so while the Delian League turn out to be long-established, the reputation quo of a comparable league develop available to ensure Sparta's safety. There were different metropolis-states that Sparta turn out to be enemies with, which encompass the Argives, who held a exceptional deal of energy themselves. As such, the Peloponnesian League have turn out to be established out of necessity rather than that of desire for war and energy over others.

Who Joined the Peloponnesian League?

Sparta turned into the leader of the Peloponnesian League in addition to its founder. The biggest members of the league (that we understand of) protected Corinth, Melos, Mantinea, Boeotia, Kythira, Pylos, Ambracia and Lefkada. There has been debates whether or now not Macedonia changed into a part of the Peloponnesian League or no longer, regardless of the truth that the overall consensus come to be that they remained impartial all through conflicts.

The Downfall of the Peloponnesian League

The Peloponnesian League commenced to fall after Sparta had out of place the struggle inside the course of Thebes at Leuktra. The Spartans had suffered brilliant lack of electricity after this war and masses of different city-states, along side Arcadia, took benefit of this and hooked up the Arcadian League. Those participants of the Peloponnesian League who stayed proper to Sparta had alternatives – both stand with Thebes or live unbiased. Around 366/5 BCE, the Peloponnesian League in the end ceased.

The Fall of Sparta

The Battle of Leuktra marked the begin of the save you for Sparta. Under the control of Epaminodas, the excellent Theban big, Thebes gained battles in opposition to Sparta at Tegyra in 375 BCE and at Leuktra in 371 BCE. These defeats took their toll on Sparta and their power waned rapid. Messenia, which have been underneath Spartan manage for hundreds of years, end up now ruled by using manner of Thebes. Sparta persisted, however they had been now not whatever but every other minor metropolis. They had fallen.

The Fight for Power

After Sparta had fallen in strength and call, there was a fight amongst Thebes and Athens as to who turn out to be to take area because the dominant power in Greece. They both desired to establish themselves to the north but might stop at not some thing to stop the opportunity from doing so. In the stop, Athens joined forces with Sparta and each faced Thebes at Mantinea in 362 BCE. While Thebes changed into splendid, their exceptional large, Epaminondas, turned into killed in battle. This brought on the waning of the Theban strength.

As a end result, there has been a electricity vacuum in Greece and there was a scramble by manner of numerous states to fill the void. Sparta, Athens and Thebes had been not in a position to persuade Greece as a united america because of numerous reasons - Sparta grow to be now not sturdy sufficient to wield such electricity, Athens have emerge as going thru issues with the Second Naval Confederacy and Thebes had out of location its first-rate well-known with no one else to take his area. It have become apparent that till there has been a person sturdy enough to manual Greece, the us of a turned into going to revert into chaos. However, inside the north of the united states of the usa, there has been the rumblings of a rustic named Macedon who end up to be sturdy sufficient to manual the Greeks to a ultra-modern technology.

Chapter 6: Famous Spartans

Sparta as a country has typically been stated for its energy however it turned into the humans themselves that made Sparta brilliant. Without certain individuals, Sparta won't have grown as wonderful as it become. The following are some of the quality and most well-known Spartans.

Famous Spartans

Arachidamia

Spartan girls have been appeared for their outstanding bodily power but Arachidamia changed into one of the most effective and bravest Spartan women. She modified into married to Eudamidas I in some unspecified time inside the destiny of the 1/3 century BCE. At the time of the siege of Lacedaemon, the Spartan Elders had decided that it became higher if the women were transported to Crete to live solid. Arachidamia, as a substitute, decided in opposition to this and jumped up, brandishing a sword in her hand and argued with the Gerousia whether or no longer Spartan ladies had been expected to live to inform the story. As a end result, Arachidamia is regularly accepted with how girls were visible in Spartan society.

Chelidonis

Chelidonis grow to be a Spartan princess, the daughter of Leotychides and the wife of Cleonymus, a man hundreds older than her. Unfortunately, she did now not stay dedicated to her husband and had an affair with Acrotatus. As a quit end result of this affair in addition to being excluded from the throne, Cleonymus invited Pyrrhus to try to triumph over Sparta. Chelidonis turned into organized to kill herself but Pyrrhus grow to be overwhelmed once more with the aid of Acrotatus.

Cynisca

Also called Kyneska, Cynisca changed into a Spartan princess, the daughter of Archidamus II. She is famous for being the primary woman to win the Olympic Games, mainly, the 4 horse chariot races, the simplest interest that women had been authorized to compete in.

Gorgo

Gorgo changed right into a queen of Sparta, the daughter of King Cleomenes I and the partner of King Leonidas I with whom she come to be the mom of the destiny King Pieistarchus. Just before the Persians invaded, Demaratus changed into stuck in Persia but despatched a timber pill covered in wax to Sparta. When it arrived, everyone turned into confused with the aid of this but Gorgo suggested that the wax ought to be eliminated, and so the warning have emerge as displayed.

Lycurgus

Lycurgus is often referred to as the lawgiver and even as he is a legendary parent, whether or not or no longer he become a historical man or woman or no longer remains a matter range quantity of debate. The foundation of the Spartan state is regularly ascribed to him, similarly to the status quo of the Gerousia, the requirement that all citizens positioned the u . S . First and that all men want to eat together to create concord.

Famous Kings of Sparta

Whereas exclusive Greek city-states have been dominated over via the use of using a single king, Sparta have become unique in that it had two. This dual monarchy became designed to preserve a stability of the political energy that leaders possessed, making sure that the u . S . And her residents is probably stored constant from one king wielding an excessive amount of strength.

The Bloodlines

The Spartan kings within the direction of the centuries were descended from bloodlines – the Eurypontids and the Agiads. Whilst these weren't the names of the primary kings, the families had been named in their honour and are believed to have emerged at the identical time in Spartan history. However, it ought to be compelled that it is impossible to ensure as to who truely dominated Sparta, specially in its early years. There are some of lists which have survived from antiquity offering the names of some kings, however whether or no longer or no longer they may be proper or were modified stays hotly contested amongst pupils.

The Agiad Dynasty

The first of the Agiad dynasty grow to be someone named Eurystene but the family line became named after the second one king, called Agis, who come to be stated to have dominated for approximately 3 a long term. He have emerge as the son of Eurstenes however received the kingship after which had the dynasty named after him.

The Eurypontid Dynasty

The Eurypontid dynasty was named after Eurypon, the 1/3 ruler of the bloodline, which emerged while the Agiad dynasty did.

Duties of the Spartan Kings

The kings had numerous roles in Spartan society. They acted because the intermediary a few of the Spartans and the gods, performing as clergymen, further to handling inner and outdoor politics and serving as judges in court docket docket. In addition to this, Spartan kings needed to be ambitious warriors themselves for after they went to warfare.

Important Kings of Sparta

Sparta changed into a robust, navy country with warriors who have been fearsome in battle, however the kings themselves had been moreover sturdy figures who formed the history of Sparta.

Leonidas

Leonidas is likely the maximum well-known Spartan king in the data of the kingdom. He changed into the leader of the three hundred warriors who unsuccessfully defended the slim bypass at Thermopylae toward the Persian invaders. He come to be believed to be round 60 years vintage at the same time as he died at Thermopylae and had been ruling along together with his co-ruler for spherical a decade.

Cleomenes I

Cleomenes ruled for round 3 a long time between the 6th and fifth centuries BCE and have become famous for his political and military techniques. He grow to be in the back of the advent of the Peloponnesian League and modified into part of the Agiad dynasty in addition to the half of of-brother of Leonidas I who traced their own family line decrease back to Hercules. In 570 BCE, he drove out the tyrant Hippias and supported the adversaries of Cleisthenes, one of the initiators of Athenian democracy. He changed into additionally recognised for his excessive love of pink wine and changed into in the long run imprisoned wherein he killed himself. His daughter, Gorgo, married his half of of-brother, Leonidas.

Archidamos II

Archidamos II come to be an Eurypontid king who dominated Sparta among 476 to 427 BCE. He have end up married twice, first to Lampito who bore him his son, Agis II, after which to Eupoleia who bore him his son, Agesilaus II and his daughter, Cynisca. He took the kingship after his grandfather, King Leotychidas, were exiled due to corruption. He delivered the surrender to the First Peloponnesian War in 446 BCE with an settlement with Pericles and the Thirty Years Peace.

Agis IV

Agis IV ruled Sparta for spherical four years on the equal time as he have become in spite of the reality that in his twenties. He have end up the 25th ruler of the Eurypontid dynasty and changed into well-known for preserving the traditions of Sparta. During the 0.33 century BCE, Sparta had forgotten the vintage strategies and Agis, thru supplying to divide his lands most of the two better ranking social education, turn out to be capable of stabilize the united states of america.

Nabis

Nabis dominated an impartial Sparta round 207 BCE till he became assassinated in 192 BCE through the Aetolian League. The last Spartan rule, he super held a small quantity of power and his lands had been quite small in assessment to earlier kings. Ancient belongings regularly mock him, portraying him as a monster by manner of the Greek historian Polybius, however that is absolutely now not the historic case. Nabis took the throne whilst the rightful heir, Pelops, modified into too more youthful to take control. In 197 BCE, Nabis turned into able to battle Argos from Philip V of Macedonia who become fighting in competition to Rome at the time. By setting a address Titus Quinctius Flaminius, Nabis changed into capable of preserve Argos. However, Flaminius proclaimed Nabis to be a tyrant and he have become forced handy over Argos to Rome.

Chapter 7: The Spartan Society

Overview of Spartan Society and Values

Sparta, now not like special Greek town-states, had a very specific social and political shape that revolved spherical its army could likely. The primary aim of Spartan society end up to deliver expert warriors who may also want to defend the united states and hold its dominance. The Spartans believed that army electricity have end up the vital issue to their survival and achievement.

Spartan society become divided into three amazing classes: the Spartiates, the perioikoi, and the helots. At the pinnacle of the social hierarchy have been the Spartiates, who've been full Spartan residents. They had been the descendants of the precise Spartan warriors who had correctly conquered and subjugated the native population of Laconia. Spartiates loved privileges and rights which have been denied to the decrease schooling.

The Spartiates were a small minority inner Spartan society, however they held extensive strength and affect. They had been the first-class ones allowed to take part in political evaluations and keep public office. The Spartiates were moreover the best of a kind individuals of the citizen armed forces, known as the hoplites, who long-established the spine of the Spartan navy.

Below the Spartiates had been the perioikoi, loose populace of Sparta who have been not taken into consideration whole citizens. The perioikoi finished a crucial position in the economic prosperity of the town-nation. They had been greater often than now not artisans, consumers, and investors who furnished essential items and offerings to Spartan society. Although they have been now not allowed to take part in the political opinions of Sparta, that they'd relative freedom compared to the helots and were covered under Spartan regulation.

At the lowest rung of the social ladder had been the helots, a country-owned slave beauty who worked the land and served the

Spartiates. The helots have been commonly agricultural employees, answerable for cultivating the land and producing meals for the Spartan citizens. However, their recognition changed into one in each of servitude, and they lived below harsh conditions. The helots outnumbered the Spartans via manner of a excellent margin, which created normal fears the various ruling class of capability uprisings or rebellions.

The Spartan society revolved spherical a strict code of conduct referred to as the eunomia. This code emphasized self-control, obedience, and the subjugation of individual dreams for the collective welfare of the kingdom. The Spartans believed that the electricity of the character grow to be ultimately measured by their contribution to the nicely-being and protection of Sparta.

The eunomia have end up ingrained in each element of Spartan existence, from schooling and education to everyday customs and rituals. The Spartans have been appeared for his or her unwavering commitment to the dominion and their capability to go through bodily hardships. They were taught from a younger age to prioritize the collective over the individual, valuing the commonplace suitable above non-public dreams.

The Spartan society's hobby on military prowess and self-sacrifice set it aside from one-of-a-type Greek metropolis-states. While Athens celebrated highbrow and creative achievements, Sparta prioritized physical power and military excellence. This singular recognition on army preparedness allowed Sparta to maintain a powerful reputation in the route of historic Greece.

Role of Kings in Sparta

The diarchy, the Spartan device of dual kingship, grow to be a extremely good feature of Spartan society. It involved kings, one from each of the 2 royal households: the Agiads and the Eurypontids. The diarchy ensured a stability of energy and authority, preventing any person person from becoming too dominant and safeguarding in opposition to capacity abuses of energy.

The kings held massive have an impact on and completed essential roles in every army and political critiques. They had been considered the embodiment of Spartan values and traditions, predicted to influence with the aid of example and cling to the stern code of conduct that dominated Spartan lifestyles.

From an early age, the kings were raised and informed along exceptional Spartan boys inside the agoge. They underwent the equal rigorous physical and intellectual schooling, enduring grueling wearing sports, combat drills, and Spartan traditions. This upbringing instilled in them the virtues of location, courage, and self-sacrifice, making equipped them for their future roles as leaders of Sparta.

In times of conflict, the kings assumed the characteristic of navy commanders. They held the authority to say battle and make vital navy options. The kings led the Spartan military into conflict, placing the example for bravery and galvanizing their infantrymen to fight with unwavering electricity of will. They were quite professional warriors themselves, main from the the front strains and risking their lives along their guys.

During peacetime, the kings had been chargeable for the manipulate of justice. They acted as judges in criminal topics, making sure the honest and equitable decision of disputes. The kings also presided over the Gerousia, the Spartan council of elders. The Gerousia consisted of 28 people, collectively with the two kings, who've been answerable for imparting and discussing laws, similarly to supplying recommendation and guidance to the ruling class.

Beyond their military and judicial roles, the kings achieved a giant feature in shaping Spartan distant places insurance. They have been liable for forging alliances, keeping diplomatic individuals of the family with distinct town-states, and representing Sparta at the nearby and international degree. The kings' capability to navigate political complexities and stable awesome alliances modified into important in safeguarding Spartan pastimes.

The position of the kings, however, become now not with out obstacles. While they held massive authority, they had been no longer absolute rulers. They were certain via the laws and customs of Sparta, and their selections had been issue to the scrutiny of the Gerousia and the broader Spartan society. The kings had to navigate the complex internet of Spartan politics, placing a touchy stability amongst their very own aspirations and the collective pursuits of Sparta.

Leonidas, as one of the Spartan kings, shouldered the weighty duties related to his role. He embodied the values of energy, courage, and self-sacrifice that have been exceedingly reputable in Spartan society. His upbringing in the agoge and his unwavering dedication to the defense of Sparta made him a herbal chief and exemplar of the Spartan ethos.

In the following economic destroy, we're able to explore the ancient context surrounding the Persian Empire and its invasion of Greece. By understanding the Persian chance confronted via manner of Leonidas and the Greek city-states, we are capable of benefit deeper insights into the importance of his control at the Battle of Thermopylae.

Chapter 8: The Persian Threat

Historical Context: Persian Empire

The rise of the Persian Empire underneath Cyrus the Great marked a huge turning detail in historic statistics. In the sixth century BCE, Cyrus released into a sequence of army campaigns that delivered about the conquest of big territories, putting in place the muse for one of the finest empires the world had ever seen. His empire stretched from Asia Minor to the Indus Valley, encompassing lands with severa cultures and populations.

Cyrus's conquests have been characterised via a tremendously lenient approach in the direction of conquered peoples, permitting them to hold their customs, traditions, and religious practices. This policy of tolerance played a critical position in keeping balance and securing the loyalty of the severa populations within the empire.

After Cyrus's loss of life, his successors, which consist of Cambyses II and Darius I, persisted to increase and consolidate the Persian

Empire. Darius I, who got here to electricity in 522 BCE, achieved administrative and economic reforms that further bolstered the empire. He set up a machine of satrapies, dividing the empire into provinces dominated with the aid of manner of satraps who amassed taxes, maintained order, and ensured the loyalty in their areas.

Under Darius's rule, the empire flourished economically. The construction of an green avenue system, known as the Royal Road, facilitated alternate and conversation all through huge distances. This community of roads associated the fundamental cities and allowed for the green movement of products and statistics in the route of the empire.

The Persian Empire boasted a powerful army stress. The Persian army comprised each professional squaddies and conscripted troops from numerous areas, resulting in a numerous combo of infantry, cavalry, and archers. The empire's military electricity emerge as similarly augmented with the resource of the use of the development of a effective military, permitting the Persians to project their power all through the Mediterranean and dominate critical exchange routes.

Xerxes I, the son of Darius I, ascended to the Persian throne in 486 BCE. He inherited an empire that turn out to be each expansive and wealthy, however he harbored a burning desire to avenge the Persian defeat at the Battle of Marathon, wherein the Greeks had thwarted a preceding Persian invasion. Determined to overcome Greece and crush any resistance, Xerxes assembled an widespread invasion pressure.

Xerxes's navy become said to amount in the loads of plenty, decided via a massive fleet of warships and supply vessels. The Persian forces have been drawn from severa regions, showcasing the empire's widespread attain and military skills. The duration and scale of the Persian invasion were extraordinary inside the historical global, with Xerxes sparing no charge to ensure his victory over the Greek town-states.

However, the Greek metropolis-states' response to the Persian invasion emerge as an extended manner from unified. While some diagnosed the upcoming danger and joined forces to withstand the Persians, others hesitated, wary of the overpowering may of Xerxes's forces. The Greek city-states located themselves at a crossroads, with the upkeep in their independence and manner of lifestyles putting inside the balance.

It have turn out to be in this context of department and uncertainty that the Battle of Thermopylae occurred. The Greeks identified the strategic importance of the slender pass at Thermopylae, wherein they could use the terrain to their advantage and keep away from the Persian improve. It changed into right here that Leonidas, the Spartan king, should grow to be a vital decide within the safety of Greece in the direction of the Persian hazard.

Xerxes' Invasion of Greece

Xerxes I, the Persian king, harbored a deep preference to avenge the previous Persian defeat on the Battle of Marathon and make bigger Persian dominance over Greece. In 480 BCE, he released into an ambitious marketing campaign to conquer Greece and bring its town-states under his rule.

Gathering a big invasion strain, Xerxes assembled an navy and army which have been exceptional of their duration and scope. The land forces consisted of squaddies drawn from numerous areas of the Persian Empire, reflecting the empire's range. Accompanying the navy changed into an outstanding fleet of warships, which include triremes, the superior struggle vessels of the time.

Xerxes modified into decided to move away not something to risk in his quest for Greek conquest. He spared no fee in outfitting his troops with the best guns, armor, and sources. His forces had been now not simplest massive but additionally nicely-geared up, reflecting the might and assets of the Persian Empire.

The Persian invasion strain set out from Asia Minor, crossing the Hellespont, a slender strait that separates Europe from Asia. This crossing modified into an fantastic engineering feat, with Xerxes ordering the development of a brief bridge of boats to move his forces across the waterway. The sight of the big Persian army crossing the Hellespont struck worry into the hearts of folks who witnessed it.

As the Persian forces superior through Thrace and Macedonia, some Greek town-states submitted to Xerxes' authority, both out of worry or a choice to are seeking out favor with the Persians. However, a number of Greek town-states diagnosed the upcoming danger and resolved to face as a good deal because the Persian invasion.

Athens, a notable Greek town-usa, emerged as a pacesetter within the resistance in opposition to Xerxes. Recognizing the want for a united the the the front, the Athenians, below the guidance of their statesman Themistocles, advised different Greek city-states to enroll in forces in the face of the Persian risk. This name to motion introduced at the formation of a Greek coalition, with numerous metropolis-states contributing troops, ships, and belongings to the purpose.

The Greeks diagnosed the significance of protecting key strategic locations in the direction of the Persian boom. One such region turn out to be the bypass of Thermopylae, positioned alongside the jap coast of Greece. This slender skip, flanked via steep mountains and the sea, supplied a herbal bottleneck that might restrict the Persian navy's improvement.

Leonidas, the Spartan king, done a pivotal role in the safety of Thermopylae. Recognizing the bypass's strategic fee, Leonidas led a contingent of 3 hundred Spartan warriors, followed through using way of soldiers from wonderful Greek city-states, to preserve the line at Thermopylae. Leonidas' popularity as a professional warrior and leader strengthened the morale of the Greek forces and stimulated self notion in their ability to face up to the Persian onslaught.

The Battle of Thermopylae have to end up the defining 2d of the Persian invasion. It become right here that Leonidas and his small however decided stress should face off toward the could probably of Xerxes' military. The conflict of cultures, strategies, and military may moreover might shape the route of records and establish the legacy of Leonidas and the 3 hundred Spartans.

As Xerxes' army approached Thermopylae, Leonidas and his Greek forces organized for the upcoming warfare. The Greeks carried out the terrain to their gain, positioning themselves at the narrowest element of the pass. They constructed a protecting wall and organized for a protective stand that might test the remedy and skill of each facets.

When the Persian forces arrived, Xerxes expected an smooth victory, given the overpowering numerical benefit his army possessed. However, he underestimated the tenacity and area of the Greek forces. The Spartans, famend for his or her navy prowess, commonplace the middle of the Greek protection and served as an belief to the alternative Greek infantrymen.

For several days, the Persians launched wave after wave of attacks on the Greek defenses, but they have been now not in a position to break thru. The Greeks, preventing with unmatched valor and backbone, held their floor, inflicting heavy casualties upon the Persian ranks. The Spartans, with their phalanx formation and expert use of spears and shields, proved to be an first-rate stress that the Persians struggled to overcome.

Despite their resilience, the Greeks faced a considerable setback while a close-by resident named Ephialtes betrayed his fellow Greeks via way of disclosing a mountain course that might pass the Greek defenses at Thermopylae. This betrayal exposed the Greek flank, compromising their function and leaving them at risk of a capability encirclement.

With their situation turning into an increasing number of dire, Leonidas made the difficult desire to brush aside maximum of the Greek forces and advised them to retreat and combat a few exceptional day. He insisted that the Spartans should live in the back of to cover their allies' withdrawal and make the final sacrifice for the cause of Greek freedom.

The final Spartans, along facet a small contingent of Thespians and Thebans who refused to desert Leonidas, prepared for his or her very last stand. They understood that their actions need to have a profound effect at the path of the warfare and the morale in their fellow Greeks. The degree emerge as set for an epic warfare the various Spartan warriors and the relentless forces of Xerxes.

In a ferocious conflict, the Spartans fought with unmatched bravery and skills. Their tightly commonplace phalanx, a protect wall of interlocked shields and lengthy spears, held agency in the direction of the Persian onslaught. They inflicted heavy casualties upon the enemy, displaying unwavering region and determination. Despite being massively outnumbered, the Spartans refused to yield, preventing to the remaining guy.

Leonidas, fame at the forefront of the Spartan protection, have end up a image of resistance and heroism. He led by way of the use of instance, inspiring his guys together along together with his bravery and unwavering remedy. In the midst of the chaos, Leonidas fell in conflict, along his comrades, however their sacrifice had a profound impact on the Persian forces.

The Battle of Thermopylae set up the exceptional bravery and resilience of the Greeks within the face of overwhelming odds. Although the Spartans and their allies had been in the long run defeated, their sacrifice sent a effective message to Xerxes and his forces. They had showed that the Greeks could not give up their freedom with out difficulty and that the Persian invasion is probably met with fierce resistance.

The Battle of Thermopylae had massive effects for the Persian invasion. While Xerxes had was hoping for a quick and decisive victory, the Greek resistance at Thermopylae had offered valuable time for the metropolis-states to rally and put together for next battles. The Greeks, inspired by way of the sacrifice of Leonidas and his warriors, channeled their strength of thoughts into next victories in competition to the Persians.

The legacy of the Battle of Thermopylae continued finally of data. The Spartan sacrifice have come to be a picture of bravery, selflessness, and unwavering willpower to a reason. Their heroic stand stimulated next generations and solidified Leonidas' location as a reputable discern in Greek and military records.

The conflict of Thermopylea

Subsection 3.1: Prelude to the Battle

Before the Battle of Thermopylae unfolded, the Greeks made strategic preparations to shield the skip closer to the imminent Persian invasion. The place surrounding Thermopylae held massive significance because of its strategic vicinity and herbal defenses, making it a excessive location for the Greek city-states to make a stand towards the Persian forces.

Recognizing the strategic price of Thermopylae, the Phocians, a Greek city-country placed in the location, took the initiative to boost the skip. They built protective partitions and fortifications, aiming to dam the Persian decorate and purchase valuable time for the Greek forces to bring together and installation their defenses.

The Phocians, properly aware of the approaching Persian invasion, identified that the slender bypass of Thermopylae presented a herbal bottleneck that could be effectively defended in competition to the big Persian military. Their efforts to aid the place had been essential in supplying a protecting gain to the Greeks.

In addition to fortifications, the Phocians applied diverse protecting measures to save you the Persian decorate. They built barricades and limitations, strategically setting them alongside the skip to restrict the improvement of the Persian forces. These protective preparations have been essential in searching for precious time for the Greek town-states to unite and prepare for the Persian onslaught.

The Greek town-states, aware of the Persian threat, understood the importance of Thermopylae as a strategic chokepoint that might stall the Persian invasion. News of the Persian forces' technique despatched ripples of trouble in some unspecified time in the future of Greece, prompting metropolis-states to evaluate their capabilities and make vital selections concerning their involvement within the safety of the bypass.

One town-us of a that identified the significance of Thermopylae come to be Sparta, renowned for its army prowess and subject. Sparta, led through the use of King Leonidas, considered the protection of Thermopylae a depend of most importance. Leonidas, recognised for his control skills and determination to the Spartan manner of life, resolved to persuade a contingent of elite Spartan warriors to protect the bypass.

Leonidas's choice to protect Thermopylae changed into not simply an act of military method but a declaration of Sparta's determination to the protection of Greek freedom. The Spartans taken into consideration themselves because the defenders of Hellenic lifestyle and values, and that they located the protection of Thermopylae as a sacred duty.

As information unfold of Leonidas and his Spartan warriors' dedication to protecting Thermopylae, different Greek town-states identified the want to sign up for forces and make a contribution to the safety try. Athens, a distinguished city-america of america, responded to the decision, sending a contingent of soldiers to beautify the Greek characteristic at Thermopylae.

The Greek metropolis-states understood the significance of group spirit and cooperation inside the face of the Persian danger. A Greek coalition started to form, with metropolis-states rallying in the returned of the motive of protecting Thermopylae. This harmony, regardless of the reality that now not without its demanding situations and variations, have grow to be a testament to the Greek town-states' shared self-discipline to resisting Persian domination.

The arrangements at Thermopylae extended beyond fortifications and navy positioning. Recognizing the need for powerful communication and coordination, the Greek forces hooked up a sequence of command and completed strategies to make certain inexperienced desire-making in the direction of the war. They diagnosed the significance of concord and area in the face of the large Persian invasion.

Furthermore, the Greeks identified that the protection of Thermopylae required not first-rate military energy however additionally ethical and mental fortitude. Various metropolis-states sent poets, musicians, and athletes to inspire and uplift the spirits of the Greek forces. Their presence provided a experience of camaraderie and reminded the soldiers of the noble motive they were fighting for.

As the Persian forces drew in the direction of Thermopylae, the Greek coalition prepared for the inevitable war. The combined forces of the Greek metropolis-states, which consist of the Spartan warriors underneath Leonidas' command, had been determined to keep the street and repel the Persian onslaught.

The stage have become set for an epic conflict of terms at Thermopylae, wherein the self-control, skill, and area of the Greek forces could be tested in the direction of the overwhelming can also of the Persian army. The safety of the pass couldn't handiest be a warfare of bodily energy but a battle of wills and a testomony to the indomitable spirit of the Greek city-states.

Subsection 3.2: Leonidas' Leadership at Thermopylae

Leonidas, the Spartan king, finished a pivotal characteristic inside the safety of Thermopylae, displaying incredible management skills and unwavering dedication to the cause of Greek freedom. His strategic alternatives, organizational skills, and the unwavering remedy he instilled inside the Greek forces had been instrumental within the splendid safety of the bypass.

Leonidas, famend for his army prowess and management developments, identified the strategic significance of Thermopylae and the important function it completed in defending Greece in opposition to the Persian invasion. With Thermopylae's narrow skip and herbal defensive advantages, he noticed an opportunity to mount a powerful resistance against the first-rate Persian military.

Assembling a contingent of three hundred elite Spartan warriors, known as the Spartiates, Leonidas led with the resource of instance, inspiring his troops through his personal braveness, strength of will, and unwavering field. The Spartans, skilled from a extra younger age within the art work of battle, were renowned for their military prowess, and Leonidas' recognition as a expert warrior and leader strengthened the morale of the Greek forces.

Leonidas understood the significance of area and harmony inside the face of the overpowering Persian hazard. He organized the Greek forces, positioning the Spartans on the leading fringe of the safety because of their famend fight abilties and unwavering area. Alongside the Spartans, squaddies from special Greek town-states shaped a united the front, fame shoulder to shoulder in competition to the Persian onslaught.

Leonidas' control extended beyond mere military strategy. He fostered a experience of camaraderie and unity the diverse Greek forces, emphasizing the noble cause they had been preventing for—the upkeep of Greek freedom and autonomy. Leonidas changed into mentioned for most vital with the resource of the use of instance, sharing in the hardships and dangers confronted via manner of his men, and instilling a revel in of duty and sacrifice in each warrior.

Prior to the struggle, Leonidas completed a series of command and easy communication channels some of the Greek forces. This organizational structure ensured inexperienced preference-making and coordination in some unspecified time inside the future of the acute stopping. By organising a hierarchy of manage, Leonidas maximized the effectiveness of the Greek safety, permitting speedy responses to converting battlefield situations.

Leonidas' strategic picks sooner or later of the Battle of Thermopylae showcased his tactical acumen and capability to make the most the protecting blessings of the terrain. Recognizing the narrowness of the pass, he located his forces to create a powerful barrier within the course of the Persian beautify. The Spartans, famend for their tightly shaped phalanx formation, provided an impenetrable wall of shields and spears that the Persian forces struggled to breach.

Leonidas' management changed into characterised thru the usage of his unwavering solve and refusal to yield to the overpowering Persian forces. Despite going thru insurmountable odds, he instilled a enjoy of indomitable spirit and determination in his troops, inspiring them to combat with unequalled valor and resilience. The Spartans, under his steerage, mounted unwavering subject and a willingness to make the last sacrifice for the motive of Greek freedom.

Throughout the Battle of Thermopylae, Leonidas proved to be a strategic and tactical mastermind. He assessed the strengths and weaknesses of each his very private forces and the Persian military, leveraging his recognise-a manner to make the maximum vulnerabilities and maximize the effectiveness of the Greek protection. His capacity to conform to changing battlefield conditions and make fast alternatives in the warmth of warfare achieved a important feature within the Greek forces' resilience and success in repelling the Persian assaults.

Leonidas' leadership additionally extended past the immediate battlefield. His presence and unwavering power of will served as a rallying point for the Greek forces, inspiring them to fight with unwavering solve. Leonidas have come to be not simplest a commander however also a symbol of Spartan and Greek harmony, embodying the ideals of courage, area, and self-sacrifice.

Despite the eventual defeat at Thermopylae, Leonidas' management and the heroic stand of the Spartans left an indelible mark on Greek information. Their selfless sacrifice and unwavering determination to shielding Greek freedom became a symbol of bravery and resilience. Leonidas' control trends and tactical prowess is probably remembered and celebrated for generations to return back.

Subsection 3.Three: The Spartan Sacrifice

The Battle of Thermopylae may want to all the time be remembered as a testomony to the Spartan sacrifice and unwavering strength of mind within the face of overwhelming odds. Despite the eventual defeat, the heroism displayed with the aid of way of the usage of the Spartans at some diploma in the war left an indelible mark on Greek records and feature become a image of braveness and resilience.

As the Battle of Thermopylae raged on, the ultimate Spartans, together with a small contingent of Thespians and Thebans who refused to desert Leonidas, prepared for their very last stand. They understood that their actions ought to have a profound impact at the direction of the struggle and the morale in their fellow Greeks. The diploma was set for an epic conflict among the Spartan warriors and the relentless forces of Xerxes.

In a ferocious war, the Spartans fought with unequalled valor. Their tightly unique phalanx, a guard wall of interlocked shields and lengthy spears, held commercial enterprise agency towards the Persian onslaught. They inflicted heavy casualties upon the enemy, showing unwavering region and backbone. Despite being extremely outnumbered, the Spartans refused to yield, fighting to the final man.

Leonidas, status at the main edge of the Spartan safety, became a image of resistance and heroism. He led with the aid of example, inspiring his men together alongside with his bravery and unwavering remedy. In the midst of the chaos, Leonidas fell in warfare, alongside his comrades, but their sacrifice had a profound impact at the very last results of the warfare.

The Spartans' unwavering determination and disciplined preventing fashion posed a big assignment for the Persian forces. The tightly ordinary phalanx, with shields interlocked and spears thrusting beforehand, created an nearly impenetrable wall of safety. The Spartans fought with calculated precision, retaining their formation and turning in devastating blows to the Persian ranks.

The Persian forces, no matter their overwhelming numbers, struggled to triumph over the Spartan protection. The relentless assaults of the Spartans inflicted heavy casualties, and the Persians placed themselves managing a decided and disciplined adversary. The bravery and unwavering remedy displayed through the Spartans inspired fear and awe in the hearts of the Persian infantrymen.

However, the Spartans' noble resistance confronted a incredible setback even as a close-by resident named Ephialtes betrayed his fellow Greeks through revealing a mountain direction that would bypass the Greek defenses at Thermopylae. This betrayal exposed the Greek flank, compromising their feature and leaving them vulnerable to a capability encirclement.

With their state of affairs turning into increasingly dire, Leonidas made the hard choice to brush aside most of the Greek forces and advised them to retreat and fight a few other day. He insisted that the Spartans may live in the returned of to cover their allies' withdrawal and make the final sacrifice for the purpose of Greek freedom.

The last Spartans, numbering round 3 hundred, along issue the small contingent of Thespians and Thebans, stood their floor and organized for the final assault. Aware in their impending destiny, they embraced their future with a revel in of obligation, honor, and the understanding that their sacrifice have to function a rallying cry for destiny generations.

In the very last moments of the battle, the Spartans fought with unmatched valor and backbone. They engaged the Persian forces with unyielding treatment, causing heavy casualties upon their adversaries. Each Spartan warrior, driven through a deep dedication to their vicinity of transport and their fellow warriors, fought with a enjoy of motive and bravado that defied the overwhelming odds stacked within the route of them.

The Spartan sacrifice at Thermopylae have end up not simply an act of determined bravery but a calculated approach to shop for time for the Greek metropolis-states to regroup and prepare for subsequent battles. Aware of the significance of stalling the Persian growth, the Spartans aimed to inflict as an awful lot harm as feasible upon the Persian forces and create a enjoy of doubt and hesitation among their ranks.

The reminiscence of the Spartans' sacrifice could reverberate all through Greece and past. Their heroic stand have come to be a picture of braveness, field, and selflessness. Their unwavering dedication to the motive of Greek freedom inspired next generations and solidified their area in facts because the embodiment of the Spartan ethos.

The Battle of Thermopylae, despite the fact that in the end a defeat for the Greeks, had some distance-engaging in consequences for the Persian invasion. The resistance displayed via way of manner of the Spartans and their allies at Thermopylae behind schedule the Persian increase and purchased treasured time for the city-states to rally and prepare for next battles. The Persian forces, although triumphant, suffered sizable losses, every in phrases of manpower and morale.

The sacrifice of Leonidas and the Spartans moreover had a profound effect at the morale of the Greek forces. The heroism displayed at Thermopylae served as a rallying cry for the Greek town-states, igniting a spirit of resistance and backbone that could deliver them to subsequent victories in opposition to the Persians.

In the aftermath of the Battle of Thermopylae, the Spartans were hailed as heroes and martyrs. Their unwavering determination, disciplined stopping style, and the sacrifice they made to defend Greek freedom have come to be legendary. Their names and deeds were all the time etched in Greek information and mythology, serving as an notion for future generations.

The Battle of Thermopylae and the Spartan sacrifice have emerge as a defining second in

Greek facts, symbolizing the resilience of the Greek metropolis-states inside the face of adversity. The unwavering self-control and bravery displayed thru the Spartans at Thermopylae maintain to captivate the creativeness and serve as a reminder of the power of sacrifice and the iconic legacy of folks who fought for the ideals of freedom and independence.

In the subsequent financial ruin, we will find out the aftermath of the Battle of Thermopylae, reading the effect of the Spartan sacrifice on subsequent occasions and the broader importance of the conflict in shaping the route of the Persian Wars.

Chapter 9: After Thermopylae

The Battle of Thermopylae marked a turning element in the Persian invasion of Greece, leaving an indelible mark on Greek history and frightening a renewed experience of willpower and concord a number of the metropolis-states. After the heroic sacrifice of Leonidas and his Spartan warriors, the Greeks faced the task of regrouping and persevering with the combat against the Persian forces.

Greek Resilience and Consolidation

In the aftermath of the Battle of Thermopylae and the heroic sacrifice of Leonidas and his Spartan warriors, the Greek town-states were faced with the sizable assignment of regrouping and continuing the fight in the route of the Persian forces. The memory of the Spartan sacrifice resonated deeply in the hearts of the Greeks, serving as a powerful concept for their ongoing warfare for freedom.

News of the Spartans' bravery and determination unfold during Greece, igniting a renewed sense of defiance and organization spirit most of the city-states. The sacrifice made through the use of Leonidas and his warriors have become a rallying cry, symbolizing the selflessness and unwavering willpower to the cause of Greek freedom.

The Greek metropolis-states diagnosed the want for harmony and coordination to efficiently confront the Persian invasion. Leaders from severa town-states convened to strategize and guide their defenses in opposition to the advancing Persian army. Despite the initial setbacks at Thermopylae, the Greeks have been decided to stand as much as the Persian forces and protect their location of beginning.

One city-united states of america that finished a essential feature in rallying the Greeks become Athens. Despite enduring the devastation of the Persian invasion and the loss at the Battle of Marathon a decade earlier, Athens emerged as a beacon of resilience and resolution. Led by way of way of statesmen which incorporates Themistocles, Athens took on a manage role in encouraging the Greek city-states to face united and hold the combat towards the Persian invaders.

Themistocles, a visionary chief regarded for his political acumen and strategic wondering, diagnosed the importance of naval strength in tough the Persian forces. He understood that the Persian military, which controlled the seas, posed a tremendous hazard to Greek independence. Themistocles advocated for the strengthening of the Greek naval forces, urging the metropolis-states to construct and contribute to a unified fleet.

The Greeks understood the want of consolidating their resources and efforts to counter the Persian invasion. Each town-united states of america contributed its military forces, financial assets, and manpower to the common cause. This collaborative technique allowed the Greeks to pool their strengths and coordinate their strategies toward the Persian forces.

The rallying cry of concord resonated all through Greece as metropolis-states set apart their differences and labored inside the path of a common purpose. The Greek town-states identified that exceptional via manner of status collectively may additionally need to they choice to face as much as the may additionally of the Persian empire.

To facilitate this concord, the metropolis-states installation alliances and everyday a loose confederation known as the Hellenic League. Led via Sparta and Athens, the league aimed to coordinate the protection efforts and collective strategies in the direction of the Persian invasion. Through this alliance, the Greek metropolis-states sought to capitalize on their individual strengths and bolster their possibilities of achievement.

The Greek city-states additionally recognized the significance of retaining the morale in their residents. They understood that the a fulfillment protection in opposition to the Persian forces required no longer truly army might likely but moreover the guide and backbone of the civilian population. Rousing speeches, patriotic songs, and public ceremonies were organized to inspire the humans and foster a sense of country wide team spirit.

Despite the setbacks at Thermopylae, the Greeks determined solace inside the fact that that that that they had succeeded in delaying the Persian improve. The heroic resistance of the Spartans, coupled with the strategic preparations made at Thermopylae and the subsequent battles, supplied the Greeks with the time they needed to regroup and consolidate their forces.

The memory of Thermopylae served as a reminder that the Persian invasion is probably resisted. The Greeks drew energy from the information that they were combating now not exceptional for his or her person city-states however for the beliefs of freedom, democracy, and the upkeep of Greek civilization.

As the Greek city-states labored within the course of consolidating their defenses, the Persian forces endured their decorate. The Greek resistance confronted in addition worrying conditions, however the reminiscence of Thermopylae remained a the use of stress, pushing the Greeks to redouble their efforts and confront the Persian invaders.

Naval Warfare and the Battle of Artemisium

As the Greek town-states regrouped after the Battle of Thermopylae, they recognized the importance of defending their coastlines and tough the Persian naval forces. The Persian Empire boasted an outstanding military, and the Greeks understood that their maritime power become critical in preventing further Persian incursions into their territories.

To counter the Persian naval hazard, the Greek city-states deployed a fleet of ships to the straits of Artemisium, a slender channel on the japanese coast of Greece. Led with the aid of the Spartan popular Eurybiades, the Greek fleet organized for a naval conflict of phrases that could play a decisive function in the outcome of the Persian invasion.

The Battle of Artemisium spread out concurrently with the activities at Thermopylae. The Greek fleet, comprising ships from numerous metropolis-states, engaged the Persian navy in a chain of excessive naval clashes. The very last effects of those battles could have a ways-attaining consequences for the Greek resistance and the Persian invasion.

The Greek fleet at Artemisium confronted a frightening task. The Persian military, underneath the command of King Xerxes, boasted a incredible armada, which include ships from severa conquered territories. The Persian fleet a ways outnumbered the Greek ships and possessed extra belongings and experience in naval war.

The battles at Artemisium have been fierce and tough-fought, with each elements inflicting heavy losses upon each other. The Greek fleet, united of their determination to guard their hometown, showcased their naval facts and maneuverability to counter the Persian forces.

The Greeks, but being outnumbered, hired strategic techniques to maximise their gain. They performed their know-how of the nearby waters, collectively with the treacherous shoreline and strong currents, to their gain. The slim straits of Artemisium furnished opportunities for the Greeks to make use of hit-and-run techniques and make the most the Persian ships' lack of maneuverability.

The Greek naval forces, constituted of triremes—speedy and agile warships with 3 rows of oars—validated their advanced maneuverability and coordination. The triremes, operated by the usage of professional rowers and prepared with a bronze ram at the bow, allowed the Greeks to execute rapid and decisive assaults at the Persian ships.

The Greek ships, forming a tightly knit formation referred to as the "line-abreast," furnished a powerful protection within the path of the Persian navy. The interlocked shields and disciplined rowing allowed for powerful coordination and protected the flanks of the fleet.

The battles at Artemisium were marked thru a chain of clashes, every facet searching for to gain the pinnacle hand. Both the Greek and Persian forces displayed bravery and resolution, carrying out fierce naval combat with their respective strengths and strategies.

Despite their numerical downside, the Greek fleet managed to repel numerous Persian assaults and keep their position at Artemisium. The naval clashes showcased the Greeks' resilience, expertise, and unwavering self-control to defending their coastlines toward the Persian invaders.

While the very last outcomes of the naval battles at Artemisium did no longer yield a decisive victory for both detail, they supplied the Greeks with a much-preferred morale growth. The Greeks proved that the Persian forces may be challenged, causing amazing losses upon the Persian army and demonstrating their naval prowess.

The Battle of Artemisium additionally served as a strategic delaying tactic, buying valuable time for the Greeks to decorate their defenses and in addition prepare for next battles. The fierce resistance and the Greek fleet's ability to hold their floor prevented the Persians from making massive improvement along the jap coast of Greece.

The achievements of the Greek fleet at Artemisium set the diploma for the decisive naval engagement that would take region later—the Battle of Salamis. The naval clashes at Artemisium boosted the self perception and morale of the Greek forces, solidifying their remedy to confront the Persian invaders head-on.

The Battle of Artemisium showcased the significance of naval strength and highlighted the Greeks' naval facts. It showed that the Persians, however their overwhelming numbers, will be efficiently challenged and repelled by way of the use of using the ability and determination of the Greek naval forces.

The Fall of Athens and the Battle of Salamis

While the Greek fleet fought valiantly at Artemisium, the Persian land forces endured their increase, primary to the fall of Athens. The Athenians, privy to the impending destruction, evacuated their town, searching out safe haven on the nearby island of Salamis. The diploma modified into set for a pivotal naval disagreement—the Battle of Salamis.

As the Persians laid siege to Athens, the Greek metropolis-states converged at Salamis to strategize their subsequent pass.

Themistocles, the Athenian statesman, finished a vital characteristic in shaping the Greek response. Recognizing the strategic importance of naval warfare, Themistocles encouraged for a decisive naval war within the path of the Persians.

Themistocles' approach targeted at the Greek fleet's functionality to confront the Persian military. He understood that the Persian forces relied closely on their naval supremacy, and with the aid of difficult and defeating the Persian fleet, the Greeks must substantially weaken the Persian invasion.

The Battle of Salamis could turn out to be one of the maximum big engagements of the Persian Wars. The Greek fleet, which embody ships from severa metropolis-states, organized to stand the Persian military in a warfare of phrases that would decide the destiny of Greece.

Led with the beneficial resource of Themistocles and united by using manner of the usage of a common desire to guard their area of beginning, the Greek fleet located itself close to Salamis, taking benefit of the slender straits that furnished a strategic gain. Themistocles orchestrated a ruse to trap the Persian fleet into the confined waters, wherein their numerical superiority might be negated.

As the Persian fleet advanced into the slim straits, the Greek ships maneuvered skillfully, launching a coordinated attack on the Persian navy. The Greek triremes, with their agility and velocity, outmaneuvered the bigger, much less nimble Persian vessels, setting them with devastating impact.

The Battle of Salamis have turn out to be characterised with the aid of the use of immoderate naval combat. The Greek ships, with their disciplined rowers and professional fighters, displayed great willpower and expertise. They used their bronze rams to ram into the Persian ships, inflicting vast harm and sinking severa vessels.

The Greek naval tactics have been designed to make the maximum the Persian military's loss of mobility inside the slim straits. The tightly packed Persian ships struggled to transport effectively, making them at risk of the precision assaults of the Greek triremes. The Greeks used their superior naval technique and coordination to their benefit, successfully breaking the Persian naval dominance.

As the battle raged on, the Greeks fought with renewed power and determination. The reminiscence of Thermopylae and the resilience displayed by using manner of Leonidas and his Spartans served as a rallying cry, inspiring the Greek forces to push forward and confront the Persian invaders.

The Greek naval victory at Salamis dealt a severe blow to Xerxes' invasion plans. The lack of a great a part of the Persian fleet undermined the Persian forces' capacity to preserve their advertising and marketing advertising and marketing marketing campaign and threatened their time-commemorated function in Greece.

The Battle of Salamis marked a turning difficulty in the Persian invasion. It tested that the Persians have been not invincible and that the Greek city-states possessed the ability, resilience, and determination to project and repel their formidable foe.

The aftermath of the Battle of Salamis noticed the Greeks celebrating a tough-fought victory. The Persian forces, shaken via their defeat, confronted a massive setback of their advertising campaign. The Greek metropolis-states, buoyed through their fulfillment, solidified their dedication to the purpose of shielding their freedom.

The victory at Salamis have become now not only a army triumph but moreover a morale booster for the Greek forces. It tested the power of concord and strategic making plans. The Greek metropolis-states, as quickly as fragmented and divided, had come collectively to stand a commonplace enemy and emerge remarkable.

The Battle of Salamis furthermore had a profound effect on the Greek city-states' perception of their private competencies. The defeat of the Persian army showcased the Greeks' naval facts and prowess, instilling a revel in of self belief and reinforcing their determination to guard their area of origin.

The importance of the Battle of Salamis reverberated a ways past Greece. The Persian defeat changed right into a blow to the strong Persian Empire, which had previously appeared unstoppable in its conquests. The Greeks had no longer most effective defended their freedom however moreover dealt a severe blow to the Persian forces, shaping the direction of records.

The Greek naval victory at Salamis paved the way for subsequent successes within the Persian Wars. It boosted Greek morale, stimulated in addition resistance, and set the degree for the very last decisive engagements that would have a examine.

The Aftermath and Legacy

The Persian Wars, marked with the useful resource of heroic sacrifices and decisive victories, left a profound impact on Greece and its legacy in shaping the route of Western civilization. The aftermath of these conflicts saw the Greeks emerge effective, defending their freedom and retaining their cultural identity in competition to the sturdy Persian Empire.

The Greek metropolis-states, united by means of a not unusual motive, persevered their resistance in competition to the Persian forces following the victories at Salamis and Plataea. The Persian invasion, while no longer absolutely halted, suffered large setbacks, and the Greeks stood company in their strength of mind to protect their autonomy and way of life.

The Greek victories inside the Persian Wars marked a turning aspect in global history. The triumph of Greek civilization over the targets of the Persian Empire mounted the strength of democracy, person valor, and navy capability. It installed the Greeks as a powerful force and laid the muse for the subsequent improvement of Western civilization.

The aftermath of the Persian Wars witnessed the Greek city-states reaffirming their commitment to the ideals of freedom and democratic governance. The victories towards the Persians instilled a experience of pleasure and self belief some of the Greeks, reinforcing their belief of their very personal cultural superiority and setting the diploma for the flourishing of Greek arts, literature, and philosophy.

One tremendous final results of the Persian Wars have become the elevation of Athens because of the fact the main metropolis-state of Greece. Athens, having performed a crucial position inside the victories at Marathon, Salamis, and Plataea, emerged as a political and cultural powerhouse. The town-us of a professional a Golden Age, characterised by manner of using the flourishing of arts, form, and philosophical notion.

The victories in opposition to the Persians additionally solidified Athens' democratic government as the version for the Greek city-states. The Athenian democracy, with its emphasis on citizen participation, equality, and freedom of expression, have end up an notion for subsequent democratic actions in the course of records.

The Persian Wars also had profound implications for the improvement of military strategies and battle. The Greeks' revolutionary use of the phalanx formation, with tightly organized ranks of carefully armored infantry, proved pretty powerful in the direction of the Persian forces. The victories at Marathon, Thermopylae, and Plataea showcased the strength of disciplined infantry, inspiring destiny navy leaders and shaping the strategies of later conflicts.

Furthermore, the Greek naval triumphs at Artemisium and Salamis confirmed the significance of naval electricity and the impact it can have at the outcome of large-scale conflicts. The Greek naval strategies, which embody using triremes and hit-and-run maneuvers, set a precedent for naval conflict and triggered next naval strategies inside the route of the historical worldwide.

The Persian Wars left a long lasting legacy inside the realm of literature and historiography. The conflicts were chronicled thru tremendous Greek historians along side Herodotus and Thucydides, who meticulously recorded the sports and provided valuable insights into the motives, techniques, and results of the wars. These historic debts function primary resources for our understanding of the Persian Wars in recent times.

The reminiscence of the Persian Wars remained deeply ingrained in Greek manner of lifestyles. The heroic sacrifices made with the useful resource of Leonidas and his Spartans at Thermopylae, the victories at Marathon and Salamis, and the collective attempt of the Greek town-states in protective their freedom have turn out to be iconic symbols of bravery, resilience, and the pursuit of noble beliefs.

The Persian Wars additionally had a profound effect on the broader ancient worldwide. The defeat of the Persian Empire shattered the perception of Persian invincibility and despatched ripples at a few stage within the japanese Mediterranean and past. The Greek victories paved the manner for a new balance of power and brought about the geopolitical panorama of the location.

The legacy of the Persian Wars extended beyond the ancient worldwide and keeps to form the modern understanding of records and way of existence. The conflicts and the values they represented have grow to be touchstones for the development of Western civilization, inspiring next generations with notions of freedom, democracy, and the pursuit of understanding.

The Persian Wars laid the foundation for the emergence of Hellenistic way of life, which may additionally unfold in the course of the japanese Mediterranean and affect the artwork, literature, and philosophy of next civilizations. The ideals of historic Greece, such as the pursuit of facts, innovative expression, and democratic governance, may come to be cornerstones of Western civilization.

The enduring legacy of the Persian Wars may be visible within the continued fascination with the conflicts in famous manner of lifestyles, which encompass literature, movie, and paintings. The Battle of Thermopylae, mainly, has captured the imagination of storytellers, who've celebrated the heroism and sacrifice of Leonidas and his Spartans in numerous creative mediums.

In surrender, the aftermath of the Persian Wars saw the Greek metropolis-states emerge effective, protecting their freedom and keeping their cultural identification in competition to the Persian Empire. The conflicts left a profound effect on Greece and its legacy in shaping the direction of Western civilization. The victories towards the Persians solidified the Greeks' belief in their non-public cultural superiority and hooked up them as an excellent strain within the historic international. The Persian Wars stimulated army techniques, inspired creative and highbrow endeavors and left a protracted lasting legacy of freedom, democracy, and the pursuit of noble ideals.

Chapter 10: Leonidas The Warrior King

Leadership Qualities of Leonidas

Leonidas, the renowned Spartan king, possessed a superb set of management tendencies that set him apart as a warrior king. His great manipulate abilities finished a pivotal role in shaping the final effects of the Battle of Thermopylae and earned him an extended lasting area in records.

One of Leonidas' maximum extraordinary control characteristics became his unwavering willpower to his human beings and his place of origin. He exemplified the Spartan first-class of setting the dreams of the country above personal dreams. This selfless strength of mind fostered a deep sense of loyalty and undergo in thoughts amongst his fellow Spartans, who observed him with utmost loyalty and devotion. Leonidas embodied the epitome of self-sacrifice, epitomizing the Spartan ethos of obligation and honor.

Leonidas changed into additionally stated for his unwavering braveness and fearlessness in the face of adversity. He displayed a steadfast willpower to shield his people and uphold their manner of life, even inside the face of overwhelming odds. This fearlessness stimulated his infantrymen and instilled in them the belief that victory have grow to be possible, no matter the challenges they faced. His braveness served as a beacon of desire and resilience for his troops, empowering them to fight with unwavering willpower.

Another super management super of Leonidas have become his ability to persuade via instance. He in no manner requested his infantrymen to do a little factor he have become no longer inclined to do himself. He fought facet with the useful resource of using issue along collectively with his guys, managing the identical risks and hardships, and his presence on the battlefield served as a rallying aspect for his troops. By principal from the frontlines, Leonidas instilled self notion in his infantrymen, assuring them that their king grow to be completely dedicated to the purpose and willing to proportion of their sacrifices.

Furthermore, Leonidas possessed a keen strategic mind and the ability to make rapid and decisive alternatives within the midst of struggle. He understood the significance of adapting to converting conditions and emerge as not afraid to adjust his approaches to advantage a bonus. His strategic acumen and short wondering were crucial in guiding his troops and maximizing their effectiveness at the battlefield. Leonidas become identified for his functionality to research complicated conditions and devise present day solutions, showcasing his strategic brilliance.

Spartan Military Training

Leonidas' first-rate control skills were cultivated through the rigorous military training that Spartans underwent from an early age. The Spartan education machine, known as the agoge, emphasised location, bodily endurance, and combat skillability. The agoge provided Leonidas with the vital tools to become an outstanding chief and warrior.

From childhood, Leonidas changed into immersed in a way of lifestyles that located a pinnacle elegance on martial excellence. He received in depth schooling within the use of weapons collectively with the spear, sword, and defend, turning into gifted of their use. The reason of this education modified into to create a substantially disciplined and green warrior beauty that might guard Sparta and its pursuits. Leonidas mastered the art of combat, developing superb capacity and precision in the use of weapons.

The agoge furthermore instilled in Leonidas a robust experience of camaraderie and teamwork. Spartan society located outstanding emphasis on the collective nicely-being of the state, and this spirit of harmony was fostered through education bodily games and communal residing. Leonidas developed deep bonds together along with his fellow trainees, forging a sense of brotherhood and shared cause that might serve him properly in the heat of warfare. This camaraderie and concord among Spartans had been instrumental of their effectiveness as a preventing pressure.

Physical fitness became some other cornerstone of Spartan navy schooling, and Leonidas excelled on this detail. Spartans had been subjected to grueling physical challenges, such as prolonged marches, immoderate exercising regimens, and competitive sports. This bodily conditioning ensured that they have been able to enduring the hardships of war and keeping their electricity and agility in fight. Leonidas, via his relentless willpower to bodily health, have become a paragon of Spartan athleticism.

The agoge additionally emphasized highbrow resilience and place. Leonidas and his fellow Spartans were professional to rise up to ache, trouble, and adversity with out succumbing to fear or melancholy. They had been taught to preserve composure below excessive pressure, permitting them to make sound picks and execute techniques correctly. This intellectual fortitude, instilled in Leonidas thru years of rigorous training, accomplished a critical characteristic in his capacity to steer with clarity and cause at the battlefield.

Battle Tactics and Strategies

Leonidas' tactical acumen and functionality to plot effective strategies had been instrumental within the success of his navy campaigns. His know-how of the strengths and weaknesses of his very own forces, as well as the ones of his adversaries, allowed him to maximise his opportunities of victory. Leonidas' strategic brilliance set him apart as a draw close tactician.

One of Leonidas' top notch techniques modified into the usage of the phalanx formation. The phalanx, a tightly packed formation of closely armored infantry, supplied a powerful wall of shields and spears that emerge as tough for the enemy to penetrate. This formation allowed for coordinated movements and provided mutual help and protection for the soldiers. Leonidas expertly hired the phalanx formation to preserve the street toward the Persian forces at the Battle of Thermopylae. By using the phalanx, Leonidas ensured that his troops furnished a united the front, with every soldier strolling in harmony to create an impenetrable safety.

Leonidas moreover recognized the importance of choosing favorable battlefield terrain. At Thermopylae, he decided on a slender bypass that confined the Persian navy's numerical benefit and negated their superior cavalry. By positioning his forces on this strategic vicinity, Leonidas minimized the impact of the Persian numerical superiority and maximized the effectiveness of his very own troops. The cautious preference of the battlefield allowed Leonidas to manipulate the float of the war and take benefit of the blessings of the terrain.

Furthermore, Leonidas understood the price of wonder and deception in struggle. He used strategic feints and fake retreats to entice the enemy into excessive wonderful positions, exploiting their overconfidence and allowing his forces to strike at critical moments. This mastery of mental conflict proved instrumental inside the successes of his navy campaigns. Leonidas employed strategic maneuvers to confuse and disorient the enemy, capitalizing on their missteps and gaining the better hand.

Leonidas' tactical brilliance prolonged past the battlefield. He possessed a keen knowledge of logistics, making sure that his troops have been properly-provisioned and equipped for the goals of warfare. He meticulously planned deliver routes and coordinated the motion of his forces, making sure that they remained agile and prepared for motion.

In addition, Leonidas possessed first-rate verbal exchange and management abilties. He had the ability to supply his orders really and concisely, ensuring that his troops understood their goals and finished their obligations with precision. His charismatic control inspired loyalty and consider among his soldiers, fostering a enjoy of group spirit and cohesion on the battlefield.

In precis, Leonidas' management trends, honed via Spartan military schooling, and his strategic acumen in conflict strategies and techniques finished a pivotal characteristic in his fulfillment as a warrior king. His unwavering dedication to his people, fearlessness within the face of adversity, and capability to manual thru instance stimulated his troops and ensured their loyalty and strength of thoughts. Leonidas' tremendous leadership and tactical brilliance hold to inspire and characteristic a testomony to the enduring strength of control and bravado.

Chapter 11: The Spartan Legacy

Spartans in Popular Culture

The Spartan legacy has had a profound impact on famous manner of existence, captivating the imaginations of humans spherical the arena. The Spartan warriors, with their fierce discipline, unwavering bravery, and commitment to the nation, have grow to be iconic figures in literature, movie, and special sorts of media.

One of the most first-rate portrayals of Spartans in popular life-style is Frank Miller's picture novel and its subsequent film model, "3 hundred." The tale recounts the Battle of Thermopylae, showcasing the valor and resilience of Leonidas and his 3 hundred Spartan warriors. The image novel and movie have become synonymous with the photograph of Spartan warriors, depicting them as indomitable heroes who fought in competition to overwhelming odds.

The reputation of "300" and similar portrayals of Spartans in media has delivered renewed interest to their stoic bravery and army prowess. The picture of the Spartan warrior, clad in bronze armor, bearing a spear and protect, has become an prolonged lasting image of courage and resilience. These portrayals have inspired infinite humans and encouraged their perception of what it manner to embody the Spartan spirit.

Beyond "300," the Spartan legacy keeps to persuade literature and film. Historical fiction novels, which consist of Steven Pressfield's "Gates of Fire," delve into the lives of Spartan warriors and offer a colourful portrayal in their training, camaraderie, and unwavering loyalty. These works of fiction seize the essence of the Spartan ethos and convey the arena of historic Sparta to life for current audiences.

In addition to literature, Spartans were featured in severa films and tv series. Their disciplined manner of lifestyles and prowess in warfare have made them popular subjects for epic recollections of heroism and sacrifice.

These portrayals often highlight the intense schooling, camaraderie, and unwavering loyalty among Spartans, taking pictures the creativeness of visitors and showcasing the long-lasting fascination with their legacy.

Influence on Military Strategies

The Spartan army techniques and strategies have additionally left an extended-lasting effect at the artwork of war. Their disciplined technique to battle and emphasis on training and steering have been studied and emulated with the resource of navy leaders at some point of data.

The phalanx formation, perfected via the Spartans, have become the backbone of many historic Greek armies. This tightly packed formation, with soldiers interlocking their shields and offering a wall of spears, furnished a effective protection and allowed for coordinated actions on the battlefield. The phalanx formation became discovered and tailored via next civilizations, demonstrating the lasting have an effect on of Spartan navy strategies.

The Spartans' emphasis on bodily fitness and conditioning also encouraged military schooling. Their notion that a robust body modified into important to fulfillment in battle resonated with later army leaders who diagnosed the significance of physical prowess in combat. Physical training and staying energy have turn out to be essential components of military training and coaching. The Spartans' interest on bodily health set a popular for future generations of warriors, inspiring the improvement of education applications that prioritize strength, persistence, and agility.

The instructions of area and unwavering loyalty instilled thru the Spartans have also unique military doctrines. The Spartan self-control to the dominion above private dreams, the strict code of behavior, and the unwavering obedience to authority had been studied and completed with the useful resource of severa navy businesses. The Spartan instance keeps to encourage leaders to domesticate area and a experience of responsibility amongst their troops. The concept of selfless carrier and setting the project above personal benefit echoes the Spartan ethos and stays a cornerstone of military control.

The emphasis on preparedness and meticulous planning, as seen in Spartan navy strategies, has moreover inspired army operations. Spartan commanders diagnosed the price of strategic questioning, intelligence accumulating, and logistical making plans. These ideas of preparedness and interest to element have fashioned the behavior of army campaigns and live vital to military techniques.

Lessons Learned from Leonidas' Leadership

The leadership of Leonidas offers treasured instructions that increase past the battlefield and stay applicable in numerous domain names of existence.

One of the vital trouble commands from Leonidas' control is the significance of most important through example. By preventing along his squaddies and sharing in their sacrifices, Leonidas stimulated unwavering loyalty and devotion. Leaders these days can studies from his instance by using manner of actively collaborating inside the demanding situations faced via their institution individuals, demonstrating dedication and selflessness. This fingers-on technique fosters a sense of brotherly love, builds receive as genuine with, and inspires others to conform with with unwavering dedication.

Another lesson from Leonidas is the significance of unwavering strength of mind and resilience. In the face of overwhelming odds, he refused to go into reverse and showed unwavering remedy. This determination inspires leaders to persevere inside the face of adversity, motivating their agencies to triumph over barriers and strive for excellence. Leonidas' unwavering willpower serves as a reminder that brilliant achievements are regularly born out of steadfast perseverance and a refusal to accept defeat.

Leonidas' strategic acumen gives some other critical lesson. He understood the strengths and weaknesses of his very very own forces and those of his adversaries, allowing him to extend effective methods and strategies. Leaders can exercising this lesson by means of way of very well assessing their institution's competencies and the aggressive landscape to make informed options and adapt their technique therefore. The functionality to analyze the situation, assume disturbing conditions, and regulate strategies for this reason is a critical issue of powerful manage.

Furthermore, Leonidas' unwavering determination to his humans and their manner of lifestyles serves as a reminder of the importance of reason-driven control. Leaders who are deeply committed to their organisation's challenge and the well-being in their organization contributors foster a feel of motive and inspire greater energy of will and loyalty. By aligning their actions with a higher reason and instilling a revel in of shared challenge, leaders can initiate their businesses to gain excellent consequences.

Additionally, Leonidas' functionality to live calm and make speedy options in excessive-pressure situations demonstrates the value of composure and easy questioning. Leaders can gain from cultivating emotional intelligence and the potential to make sound judgments below stress, fostering a enjoy

of take into account and self belief among their groups. This capability to preserve a degree head and offer regular steerage in some unspecified time within the destiny of tough instances is an indicator of powerful control.

In stop, the Spartan legacy has left an indelible mark on well-known way of life, army strategies, and control ideas. Spartans have become enduring symbols of braveness and area, fascinating audiences through diverse kinds of media. Their military strategies, collectively with the phalanx formation, keep to steer war procedures. From Leonidas' management, we analyze the importance of primary thru instance, demonstrating dedication and resilience, making strategic picks, and fostering a revel in of motive-driven leadership. The Spartan legacy serves as a reminder that the requirements of area, loyalty, and unwavering self-discipline are timeless and hold to form our understanding of manipulate and braveness.

Chapter 12: the Beginnings of the Spartan Empire

The Spartans have echoed in the course of the some time as some of the deadliest and most skilled squaddies in their time. From their ruthlessness to their functionality at the battlefield, they have been feared with the aid of most and had been unruly toward them as properly. They were said for having a political foundation which have emerge as is very unusual, now not best in our day however theirs as properly. The charge of their legends and legacy have grow to be that they lacked the humanity that makes us humans. They were bred to be the apex race, the final form of human. The Spartan Empire became said to had been a sensible response in the times of melancholy and unusual activities.

Although powerful and widely recognized, The Spartan Empire did no longer last as long as some may additionally believe to of idea. Though it end up one of the longest in its time, this become a time of numerous brief-lived empires. Sparta changed into believed to of been a completely strict, militaristic dictatorship, but it changed into now not as severe as different books tell us. They had lifestyle institutions in the course of the metropolis together with a theatre and arenas for wearing activities. Most of their manner of existence, but, changed into based on very athletic and sporty types of sports activities. Many different buildings of their society sought to be cultural thru army training.

The starting of the Spartan Empire may be very hard thus far due to the blended information that has arisen through the years. Some historians even doubt that fact that early Sparta ever existed. Many are beginning to consider that Sparta have end up once part of the Mycenaean Empire. In both actual texts and memories collectively with the "Illiad" mentions that the ruler of Sparta have become Agamemnon, brother of the King of Mycenae. Although there can be speak of a primary invasion through the Dorians round

1100BC, we do no longer truely understand. Most of the historical files, manner of life, and legends were destroyed, which left many factors of the civilization and their timeline in the unknown.

Sometimes later, Dorians came in and commenced to installation settles in Peloponnese a and Lakonia. They quick unfold out and determined colonies inside the Aegean Islands and Gortyn.

The most accurate date of setting the origins of the town of Sparta is round 850BC, and this is although confused by way of taking or deliver some years of the time. They were decided as a polis because the four cities in the vicinity united to come to be what we now comprehend due to the fact the town of Sparta, or what is likewise referred to as Lakedaemon. The small united states endured to develop up until approximately 736BC until a the First Messenian War took place. However brief it might had been, the battle changed into in the Spartans want. They conquered the Messenia state, in which the human beings had been then enslaved and given the equal remedy as the earlier said Spartan united states of america. They had been made slaves and given to the decision of helots, which means that they had been slaves, best they have been allowed advantageous privileges, some thing slaves of the time have been no longer familiar with. One not unusual misconception is that slaves of this era had been poorly handled and used to the worst of situations. This was now not the case. There were more alongside the traces of bad citizens, and that they have been blanketed within the population, which made up maximum of the country. Slaves had been not regarded down upon and had been even reputable and revered through their masters. However, the slaves did no longer maintain the same charity for his or her masters. They did not bear in thoughts the Spartan ruling and the manner they have been taken preserve of.

Tensions had constantly been immoderate, but rapid, the Messenia slaves have been no longer to tolerate the Spartan rule any longer. They in grew to grow to be revolted in competition to the Spartans and had been fast defeated, and their fame of helots have become reduced in addition. This, in flip, released severa lands given to them back to the Spartans, which have emerge as very welcomed due to the growing length in their army. The helots did no longer give up there. Over time, there had been severa revolts wherein left the Spartan Empire in a standstill. Unable to relaxation and increase in-amongst wars, tensions remained excessive with the helots, and it left the empire is a inclined nation.

Nearby, the winning usa of america of Argos become turning into ever extra adversarial in the path of the Spartan Empire. Soon enough, conflict had broken out a number of the 2, and the Argive navy have come to be actually as ambitious due to the fact the Spartan Empire. Ruthlessly, the Spartans devastated the land within the Argos Province. They were aided with the aid of the small metropolis of Asine. Feeling betrayed by way of way of the Asinians, Argos, in revenge, sacked the small city and destroyed everything, collectively with its human beings. When the Spartans turn out to be aware of this tragedy, the anxiety among the 2 states grew worse. During this time of struggle, the neighbouring states of Sparta and Argos commenced out to unfold and settle into nearby areas. Sparta changed into now not ignorant of those movements and changed into splendid to discover some towns of their very own. In 706BC, Sparta discovered Taras. Sparta changed into furthermore regarded during this era for their upgrades in musical arts.

By this time, the Spartan Empire, despite its skirmishes with its helots have become now one of the maximum powerful states in Greece. The town changed into seemed upon as a frontrunner at the same time as all of them met and agreed that Sparta must broaden a defensive alliance along with her neighbours. This agreement turns into known as the Peloponnesian League. If the helots are to riot yet again towards the Spartan state, the members of this league agreed that they will fight in a joint army that changed into proper now controlled with the aid of Spartan commanders. They might in all likelihood, in turn, ship troops to Sparta to useful useful resource them in opposition to any riot. In move lower again, the Spartans promised to defend the possibility states of Greece inside the possibility of a few component lousy have been to appear.

Around 650BC, the helots have been all all over again unhappy being beneath the rule of thumb of thumb of the Spartan rulings. Aristomenes took the Messenians and led a rebellion in competition to Sparta. Dedicatedly believing in oracles, the Spartan leaders were assured with the prediction that they might be excessive great. After a twenty prolonged year rebellion, which took a notable toll inside the direction of the Spartan Empire, they have been able to defeat the rebellion and subdue the humans of Messenia.

Chapter 13: Rise of the Spartan Empire

Due to the normal struggle of rebellions and rebellion, the Spartan leaders found out that it turned into time to make a alternate within the manner they lived, identifying that they had been glaringly doing a little element incorrect if they persisted to permit those tiny wars. Under the control of King Lycurgus, they drove Sparta via a whole navy reform. By this issue in time, the Spartan navy changed into despite the fact that commonplace maximum of the Greek polis, however in time, the quickly became one of the maximum well-known and intimidating army forces that had ever walked the earth. From the instantaneous they will understand what they were doing, greater younger boys were knowledgeable and conditioned to emerge as a number of the fiercest warriors that the arena had ever professional. This moreover covered many of the women, having the Spartan Empire receive as right with it is probably smart to make their women as hard as most guys from neighboring states.

If way of life is to be depended on, within the course of the iciness, boys have been not allowed to be absolutely clothed. With best a unmarried piece of garb, they had to go through the iciness as part of their relentless conditioning. For the girls, they had been endorsed to warfare each special and to take part within the sports activities sports activities of Sparta. Once a informal Archaic united states, they quick bread into one which was recounted for their army and athletic kingdom.

During this time, leaders had become so focused on protective their land; that that they had brought forth the custom of judging babies at beginning. If they had been considered a hazard, hassle, or inclined, they would be thrown proper into a gorge or left within the u.S.A. Of the usa to die from some aspect cause modified into meant for them. This quality ensured that lifestyles have become difficult and difficult for the Spartan human beings. They had been driven and skilled so relentlessly so it'd make sure that they may in no way lose manage of the Messenians once more. They were decided to hold their manage all the time. They nation had grow to be so strict in its beliefs; they even banned Spartans from eating alcohol.

Not quickly after their reform, Argos had another time introduced war to the Spartan Empire. At first, it changed into small battles that took place some of the 2, but some the essential conflicts delivered plenty extra destruction. The biggest struggle to come back returned from proper proper right here end up the Battle of

Hysai Argos emerge as critically defeated, and it grow to be considered the give up of the campaign. Argos changed into so ruined by means of this massive fall apart that Sparta did now not even need to march into the town. The fight were that lessen and dry while it had come to its

victor the Spartans. From proper here the conflict handiest continued the Spartan

Empire moved its people via Argos's lands. They soon captured Phigaleia, Hira, Pylos, and

Mothone

This changed into now not the cease of the war, in spite of the truth that, the number one of many that the Spartans should consecutively grow to be part of. The Spartans persisted to salary conflict in Tegea spherical 560BC. Having left part of their authorities set up inside the city, Argos speedy lower again for a few different conflict of their very personal. However, the 2 agreed that each different most vital warfare changed into now not a few aspect the two were prepared to deal with in the period in-between. They determined as a substitute that every aspect want to result in three hundred of their great hoplites and do war. This have turn out to be known as

The Battle Of Champions. The honor become said to be unfold most of the 2, regardless of being of the worst opposition. The conflict become presupposed to be so brutal or maybe that it ended with exhausted

Argivians and one wounded Spartan soldier. The advertising and marketing campaign ended proper right here, and that they Archive troops on the equal time as home to their town. However, the Spartan warrior grow to be filled with a lot grief and disgrace, he, in flip, killed himself. Both

sides however, claimed to be the victor, but no man or woman can also additionally ever certainly comprehend.

With plenty concept after the warfare, the Spartans decided to a latest fashion of hair ethics. This custom may also need to final for numerous years, and the men may want to permit their hair develop out very lengthy, and they had been now not allowed to have moustaches. The fine time they were allowed to lessen their hair is after a victorious struggle.

Although Argos turn out to be however to be completed with Sparta, the Spartan Empire, in 510BC in the long run created a information with the metropolis of Athens. Sparta with the useful resource of this issue in time became not eager on tyrants and held a immoderate distaste for them. During this yr, Sparta determined to head north and stress out the Athens tyrant, Hippias. It is a conflict that became quick lived.

Five years later, Sparta yet again positioned itself in each different battle with Argos. The cause for the short battle is unknown, however for the reason that states had such hatred and problems with the alternative, there might have been many motives that the 2 had lengthy past to battle. The Spartan navy had marched into Argolis, however the cutting-edge king, Kleomenes, changed into now not able to sack Argos itself. By this component in time, the Argos Army had end up careless and have become extensively guided. Later in that identical 12 months, the Spartan navy come to be capable of loathe the Argives who attempted to break out and find sanctuary in a holy grove close by. The Spartans, but, had been greater relentless than common. They endured beforehand and killed the Argives each with the useful resource of fireside, or that they had pushed them out to be slaughtered outdoor of the grove. By the time this combat have grow to be over, over -thirds of the Argives navy were ravaged, which end up spherical six thousand men. This become the largest loss Argos had ever persevered to the Spartans, and it might be considered that remaining critical struggle among the empires. To ensure they may by no means upward thrust once more, the Spartans went to Argos and killed every single male there was inside the town, ensuring they may die out over the years. For this era, this become considered a totally merciful component. Usually, a rival

s navy might probable overcome the city earlier than shifting in and slaughtering the citizens of the entire town.

As the Spartan Empire had moved right into a extra length, the location started out to emerge as confused. In the near distance, the Persian Empire changed into beginning to upward push and take control of the land. They had sent messengers to the cities of Sparta and Athens. Demanding property or in pass returned, they might be conquered. The Spartans reacted negatively towards this and killed the messengers. Enraged the Persian Empire plotted for warfare. While the climax turn out to be but to come, the Persian Empire invade Athens and Attika, in reaction to a insurrection the Greek had concerned themselves with early on.

This shift in balance set the earth on its toes. Athens had brought collectively representatives from the diverse Aegean States, on the facet of Sparta, to meet on the island of Delos to discuss a percentage that is probably in the long run known as the Delian League. For the states that had joined the league, they had been to send out boats and infantrymen out for the beneficial aid towards the Persian Empire. If the states did now not personal a large military, they'll permit contributing coins to help useful useful resource in the warfare strive. One of the most essential goals of this league turn out to be to loose up the states that the Persian Empire had previously taken again at the Aegean east coast.

With little interest, the Spartan Empire modified into no longer to keen to becoming a member of the league due to the truth Athens have become the leader of the extremely-modern Greek Alliance, seeing them as a bully for his or her strategies. At positive instances sooner or later of the league, severa states had attempted to go away, however Athens pressured them to stay in. Most of the ships had been conscripted in, and almost half of the finances added into the league were from Delos to Athens.

Whether or now not the Spartans had decided to help inside the early ranges of the warfare, Athens had made a amazing victory and defeated a fantastic portion of the Persian Army in 490BC at the Marathon Beach. Despite how worried Sparta had emerge as with the Athenian Empire, the Persians continued to grow as a chance as well.

The Persian Army had bred and gathered sufficient troops to bring on a big army that modified into supposed to invade Greece. At this aspect, the Persian Empire accelerated from India to Greece and the whole troop rely turned into near million. Although this huge range appears immoderate, a few state-of-the-art historians bear in mind that this turned into an inaccurate range. They believed the army emerge as to be around 3 hundred fifty thousand. Xerxes, taking the reins after his father, Darius I, marched into Greece with an military in comparison to the area had ever seen. This army wreaked havoc as it captured Macedon, Thrace, and Thessaly.

Sparta and Athens quickly observed out that they need to stand together to defeat the extra foe. The states created the Hellenic League, which become a assembly of Greek states with the intention of preventing the Persian Empire. Sparta, technically did now not need to assist for the meant purpose of this battle become Athens, but the Spartan King, Leonidas knew that the Persian Empire might be on their doorstep in the occasion that they have been now not stopped rapid sufficient.

The Spartan Empire sent 3 hundred of their superb troops to the Thermopylae Pass, in hopes of halting the Persian

s improvements. On the opposite end, Athens changed into capable of defeat the Persians in a naval struggle at Salamis, which helped to cut off Persian reinforcements. Afraid that the Greek

s may additionally reduce off his escape course domestic, Xerxes left his advertising campaign collectively with his major fashionable, Mardonius together along with his ninety thousand troops to take a maintain of Greece.

After

come convincing from the Athenian Empire, Sparta decided to take its forces north on a big advertising and marketing advertising marketing campaign to defeat the Persians. Under the King Pausanias, the Spartans met war with the Persians near the Theban metropolis of Plataea. After a bloody conflict that lasted for numerous days, the Spartans led the Greeks to victory and defeated the Persians, consequently saving the Greek states from the doom the Persians favored to carry.

After the first-rate warfare, the Spartans over again home seeking out a few peace and quiet; but, the Spartan facts is full of destruction and turmoil, and this changed into no exception. Sparta modified into starting to have hassle in retaining the loyalty of the Peloponnesian League. Many of the members had reformed to the democratic authorities at the same time as the Spartans had been despite the fact that principled in an oligarchy.

Trouble only persisted to develop for Sparta as an earthquake hit and crippled the city. Much of the city come to be destroyed and plenty of Spartiates, which can be the warrior residents that have been to make sure balance from within the metropolis, were killed. This left an opportunity for the helots to upward thrust once more in each other insurrection in competition to the metropolis. With heaps conflict, the Spartans had been able to keep off the helots at Mount

thome

but they were no longer able to keep their electricity and defeat them. Sparta quickly reached out to their allies in hopes of assist.

Athens have end up generous sufficient to send useful useful aid wherein protected a small navy, but Sparta end up not stimulated with their outreach. For a few unknown cause, Sparta declined Athens resource and refused to apply them of their marketing campaign to take another time the town. It can also were a because of a political distinction because Athens had in fact brought and have come to be presently processing an intensive democracy. To Sparta, this modified into enormously offensive because it changed into now not properly perfect with an aristocratic arch type they lived off of. This stone on the street proved to interrupt the repairing dating Sparta had with

Athens

and it left lead Athens to mistrust the Spartan Empire.

Not lengthy after, Athens soon reached out to 2 states who have been against Sparta, in an attempt to create an Alliance in competition to them. Over this time of conjuring, Athens had all started out out to paintings on troubles right away. Athens had usual a few extraordinary league that might be called the

Delian League, which turn out to be to make certain that Persia ought to in no way invade their place of birth again. It have emerge as commonly a naval fleet in comparison to the Pelleponesean League that Sparta currently had in region that have emerge as in most cases navy based definitely. Athens quick started out to blackmail sure allies in the choice of building a stronger empire. Their plans fast backfired as one in every of his preceding allies went to Sparta, begging for them to store Greece and launch them from the Athenian tyranny. Although reluctant in advance than the whole lot, they agreed to go to war with Athens and it

s Delian League. This result in the beginning of the Peloponnesian Wars.

Before any important warfare inside the battle, and along with earlier than the struggle even started out out, Sparta and Athens were now not on real phrases. They had engaged in severa small skirmishes that did no longer trade an entire lot after the warfare had been obtained. While Athens commanded the seas, Sparta and it

s floor troops demanded the land. Sparta grow to be generally decided outside of the gates of Athens, however Athens changed into smart to live in because, at the helm, became Pericles.

The struggle have become no longer an clean one and tended to bring about a stalemate for each additives. While the Delian League managed the numbers of troops and ships than Sparta and it

s Peloponnesian League, they were equaled thru manner of the superbly professional squaddies of Sparta and the help of many Greek states which covered Sicily.

During the

Pelloponnesian

War

s 2d 12 months, Sparta decided to invade

Attika

Those of who had fled and much of the Athenian military hailed decrease again to Athens, wherein they were protected by way of manner of its high partitions underneath the leadership of Pericles. Pericles had the Athenians take safe haven and safe haven at the back of the partitions, hoping to protect them from the ambitious Spartan infantrymen. Once all over again at another stalemate, Sparta became having a difficult time making any ground o

n

Athens. Without a proper military, they could not stand a hazard at the seas. However, on land, they had been now not capable of make it past the well-built fortress of Athens. This have become additionally the equal form of stalemate for the Athenian Empire. They had been now not capable of face the Spartan

s on the floor, and their military emerge as satisfactory bold within the water.

Soon, even though, Athens commenced out to educate a larger, and further lethal army over the path of time. Sparta started to put together in the direction of the Athenians intently skilled infantrymen, but Sparta in no way needed to swing a sword. A plague had appeared in Athens and interior a quick time, a majority of the military and residents had perished to the illness. Pericles himself became a victim of the deadly plague.

For the next numerous years, Sparta defeated Athens in almost each land struggle engaged. There had been battles but in which Athens come to be high-quality. The first changed into the Battle of Pylos and the second grow to be The Battle of Cythera in Laconia. Despite those defeats, Sparta grow to be however capable of capture the Athenian city of

Amphilopolis

even as crushing Athens defences within the method. Due to the regular stalemates and in no way completing bloodshed the two states decided to signal a peace treaty that have emerge as known as the Peace of Nicias. This deal modified into imagined to final for thirty years relying at the popularity of the two states. Sparta become to broadly identified the Delian League, which come to be now part of the Athenian Empire and Athens have become no longer allowed to takes steps in dismantling the Peloponnesian League.

For a while, this labored out ok, however the two couldn't stay mutual all of the time. The treaty emerge as broken manner in advance than it

s due time on the same time as Athens have to now not stand aside due to the truth the Peloponnesian League persisted to move about its affairs. Athens broke the peace and pursued to make a devastating blow in opposition to Sparta. They attempted to damage Sparta

s economic companies in Syracuse. Sending a primary fleet full of professional warriors to the city, they attacked and held the top prevent for a while. However, they for some cause did now not kill them off speedy. Sparta reached out in useful resource to its allies and generals to enhance Syracuse. When they arrived, Athens preserve in town weakened and in turn that they'd to name in reinforcements of their personal. After a long-lived warfare, the Athenians had been all all over again defeated and with it, their fleet of ships changed into captured. This is called the biggest defeat the Delian League ever skilled.

With peace at the table, Sparta seemed over it and determined to counter-attack. Thankfully, because of the truth the Persians despite the fact that held a grudge in opposition to the Athenians, they began out to fund the Spartans of their quest. With this coins, Sparta changed into able to create a fleet of ships that they'll call their personal, and they alleged to invade

Attika

The Spartans had been able to marvel and overwhelm the Athenian navy, depriving Athens in their components from

the Black Sea.

With nowhere to show, Athens retreated to its partitions to bear the conflict. As sources diminished and as they have been left defenceless, they were pressured to surrender to Sparta in 404BC. This is known as the start of Sparta

s primary strength age and the cease of the Athenian/Delian League.

Chapter 14: The Prime of the Spartan Empire

At this issue in time, 404BC, Sparta have become now

The top of their Empire. For the very last century, Greece had been in a consistent u . S . A . Of turmoil. From battle, broken treaties, betrayal, new governments, treachery, and shifts in strength, the land turn out to be in a scarred nation. Politics turn out to be becoming a top notch issue within the region, and it changed into no longer helping all through the instances of war. Sparta had in its hand the energy and energy to control this land considering that they've been at the peak of all of them. Sparta modified into nearing the issue of twenty-5 thousand citizens. They have been almost to the issue of 5 hundred thousand slaves. Persia changed into now not a chance because of a civil warfare, and Athens come to be down for the problem.

However, Sparta could not stand idle for prolonged. With a information of conflict and destruction, history could normally commonly have a tendency to duplicate itself. The Famous Ten Thousand, a famous group of Spartan infantrymen, became lead into Asia for any other conflict marketing marketing campaign instead of solidifying the Greece territory. Sparta led the struggle at some stage in Asia minor in hopes of taking down the Persian Empire, maximum probably to prevent them from ever developing to electricity again. Problems began out to stand up at the identical time as the Peloponnesian League might no longer come to Sparta

s beneficial aid. Instead, they betrayed their former member. The biggest factions to depart had been the

Thebes

and the Persians that had been as soon as an pleasant friend.

The Persian Emperor became not finished with Greece and located the correct time to strike in retaliation of the Spartan Empire. He started to send bribes to the opportunity Greek states in hopes of having them to upward thrust in competition to the Spartans. Thebes end up brief to join after which evolved an alliance with Persia. Thebes forces moved to a Spartan town, Heraclea and destroyed the city, which incorporates the slaughter of genuinely anybody there. Once listening to the facts from lower once more domestic, The Famous Ten Thousand marched another time to deal with the threat that changed into developing in Greece.

Soon the Boeotian Alliance become born. Consisting of a united pressure of Thebans, Argives, and Athenians, they campaigned in opposition to a small Spartan Army at Nemea. Despite their awesome and large army; The alliance have come to be crushed with the beneficial resource of the Spartans. This became now not the surrender, despite the reality that.

Around 377bc, thinking about the fact that Sparta had not united the Greek states, Athens had recovered from the battle and brings forth a new edition of the Delian League. One year later, the league have grow to be able to construct itself up the issue of defeating the Spartan Navy in Naxos.

In the yr of 371Bc, the struggle of Leuctra took place. Some Theban warriors had created a Greek military and fought in competition to the Spartans on the plains of Leuctra. This motion became at once due to the truth that Sparta moved in advance and captured Thebes with out provocation. This have been given the Athenians on board with the Thebans to absorb hands in competition to Sparta yet again. During this time, the Theban commander, Epaminondas, had emerge as a famous and high-quality preferred. He had created revolutionary methods that allowed the hoplites to combat with a modern-day fashion that would rival the Spartans. This machine allowed the Thebes to have more humans preventing proper now than the Spartans, who however used older army techniques. Soon enough, the 2 armies clashed and the conflict became stacked. The Spartans nevertheless had the gain. They had large numbers, properly-designed tool, and have been intently knowledgeable in their tactics. However, actually one among their biggest downfalls have become that they were proud, some factor from years of battle that had taught them. The combat emerge as so pushed, that the overall referred to as for a brief retreat. If the Spartans had retreated and regrouped, they most possibly may have received the war, however they refused to. Their honor and satisfaction as squaddies

emerge as too much and they endured to fight on. Since half of of the Spartan soldiers retreated even as others did no longer, the Theban army become able to take gain of this vulnerable factor and assault. The Spartan warriors were defeated and despatched again to retreat.

Chapter 15: The Fall of the Spartan Empire

An empire is never at its excessive for lengthy and after the defeat at Leuctra, the Spartan Empire need to never reap a higher apex. After the defeat the Spartans decrease decrease lower back to Sparta, consequently finishing the conflict. The Thebans tore down the Peloponnesian League and recreated the Boeotian League without which incorporates Sparta. As Sparta's populace had fallen because of the war in Persia and the modern-day warfare, their territories had been taken from them through using the Thebans. To upload insult to harm, Thebe than determined to loose all of Sparta's slaves and deliver them the land of Messenia to shape their country. Sparta continued to live quiet and allow the Thebans do as they desired in the direction of this time. However, Thebes quick set up the metropolis of Megalopolis north of Lakonia. This, in turn, took away all trade and change far from Sparta. This turn out to be the turning factor in which Sparta want to now not stand idly thru. They rose as plenty as regain Messenia, however they have been met with little success.

For a long time, Sparta, whether or not or not or now not forced or via manner of desire, stayed a smaller kingdom in Greece. Soon Thebes may fall, and Athens ought to all all yet again upward push to take control for a quick duration. However, blended forces of Greek states amplify up and have been defeated at the Battle of Charonea via Phillip of Macedon. With this information, the Spartans sent threats to Phillip or maybe attacked, but to their dismay, they have been defeated at the Battle of Megalopolis. This can be considered the Spartan's final foremost battle. They misplaced no land, however by no means once more may they combat in any such essential struggle.

After a few years, the son of Phillip, Alexander, had risen. He moved forward and took manage of all of the Greece except for Lakonia and Sparta. Sparta became the best u.S.A. No longer to fall below their manage. Alexander requested Sparta to help help his struggle as he marched into Persia. Some of their well-known very last phrases were, "We do not take a look at men, we lead them."

Although Alexander moved earlier, Sparta remained in a calmer state for many years, uncommon to their information of past. Staying small and to themselves, they soon could not avoid an antique time rival, Argos.

At this problem in time, the Spartan Army end up now a shadow of its former self. However, they have been despite the fact that robust. They went directly to defeat Argos numerous instances. Despite the previous information Sparta had with Argos, they were able to take the town of Argos, two instances.

After this period, the Spartans quickly positioned out of the Roman Empire that was starting to sweep the lands. Sparta turn out to be, unluckily, one of the very last cities to be captured. This become the stop of the Spartan Empire. Near the cease of the Roman

Empire, Goths stormed into Greece and destroyed what changed into left of the as soon as seemed city of Sparta.

www.ingramcontent.com/pod-product-compliance
Lightning Source LLC
Chambersburg PA
CBHW071447080526
44587CB00014B/2019